Essential Notes in Basic Sciences for the MRCPsych Part 2

WM 18

Wai-C th

Locum (

and

Kirsty

Specialis
Stockton

w/d

Radcl
Oxfor

Radcliffe Publishing Ltd
18 Marcham Road
Abingdon
Oxon OX14 1AA
United Kingdom

www.radcliffe-oxford.com
Electronic catalogue and worldwide online ordering facility.

British Library Cataloguing in Publication Data

A catalogue record for this book is available from the British Library

ISBN 1 85775 673 8

Typeset by Thomson Press (India) Ltd, Chennai, India
Printed and bound by TJ International Ltd, Padstow, Cornwall

Contents

Adults with capacity but who refuse treatment

- Treatment cannot be given to an adult who has the capacity to refuse treatment.
- Adults are presumed to be competent to refuse treatment. It is up to the health professionals to prove that the patient did not have the capacity should they decide to treat against the patient's will.
- It is good clinical practice to ask patients to sign a statement that they refuse to receive the treatment offered and accept responsibility for the potential consequences.

Adults who lack capacity

For adults who lack capacity, treatment may be given without consent under the following 3 circumstances – the first 2 are particularly relevant to the Accident and Emergency setting.

1. *Doctrine of 'necessity'*
   Doctors have a duty to treat an adult to save lives or to prevent serious harm if he or she lacks capacity to consent or refuses the proposed treatment.
2. *Mental Health Act*
   - The Mental Health Act 1983 allows patients with mental disorders to be compulsorily admitted to hospital for assessment and treatment of their mental disorders.
   - This includes treatments ancillary to the core treatment of the mental disorders but not unrelated physical disorders (B vs Croydon HA, 1995).
3. *Court's judgement*
   - Although no one can give legally valid consent on behalf of an adult who lacks capacity to give consent to proposed treatments, the High Court can make a declaration that such treatments are not unlawful.
   - This procedure can be used for cases such as sterilisation in a person with intellectual disability or proposed Caesarean section of a woman who refused the operation due to mental illness.

Patients with mental disorder

Physical treatment unrelated to underlying mental disorders
   - E.g. patients with chronic schizophrenia brought to the emergency department with a suspected myocardial infarct and who refuse appropriate emergency treatment (e.g. ECG monitoring, thrombolysis).

- The Mental Health Act is not applicable.
- Clearly, the doctor should persuade the patient to receive appropriate treatment, giving full explanations to the patient with the assistance of relatives.
- Should these measures fail, the doctor should quickly assess the patient's capacity to refuse the specific treatment for the suspected myocardial infarct.
- The more serious the consequences for non-treatment, the greater the capacity required to refuse treatments (Re T, 1993).
- If the patient lacks capacity, emergency and life-saving treatment can be given under the 'necessity doctrine'.

Direct treatment for the patient's mental disorders
See mental health law below.

Restraint and seclusion

Preventative actions

The need for restraint and seclusion may be reduced by

- adequate explanations to patients about their treatment,
- adequate personal space for patients,
- structured in-patient activities.

Restraint

- Aims to minimise unacceptable behaviour.
- Used only as a last resort and its use should be reviewed regularly.
- Staff should be trained in the techniques of restraint.
- Hospital staff have the power of reasonable restraint of formally detained patients under MHA 1983 (contains immunity from legal claims introduced by the Lunacy Act 1890).
- Power of reasonable restraint over informal patients depends only on common law rights (of self-defence, preventing a breach of peace or preventing a crime).
- If restraint is required on informal patients, detention under the Mental Health Act should be considered.
- Note that a combination of restraint and antipsychotic medication may cause acute stress and cardiac arrest.

the incompetent person and act if he or she were to experience a temporary return to capacity).
- Applications may be made by a receiver, an applicant for the appointment of a receiver, a person expected to be provided for by the incompetent person, or an attorney acting under an Enduring Power of Attorney.
- A formal hearing is held.
- Once the will is signed by the court staff, it is as valid as if it were made by the patient.

Testamentary capacity

- The capacity of a person (i.e. the testator) to make a will.
- According to Banks vs Goodfellow (1870), the testator must have the soundness of mind and memory, and understand
  - what a will is and what its consequences are,
  - the amount and value of the property he or she has, and
  - who can reasonably expect to have a claim to the property.

Powers of Attorney, Enduring Powers of Attorney

Powers of Attorney

- A legal document signed by the donor (or grantor) which gives another person (i.e. the 'attorney') the authority to make certain decisions specified in the document on behalf of the donor.
- Only matters relating to the properties and affairs of the donor are covered. The attorney cannot make personal decisions for the donor.
- The attorney can cease to act only by giving notice to the donor.
- It operates entirely in the private law of agency without intervention of the State.
- The effect is as if the decisions made by the 'attorney' were those of the donor.

Enduring Powers of Attorney

- Different from regular Powers of Attorney in that
  - The power is intended to continue in the event of subsequent mental incapacity of the donor.
  - It must be registered when the donor is or is becoming incapable.

- ○ The Court of Protection then monitors the attorney to ensure that the power is carried out consistent with the donor's original wish.
  - ○ The power may not be modified by the donor after registration.
  - ○ The power can only be revoked by the Court.
  - ○ The attorney cannot cease to act without notice to the Court.
- To be valid, the Enduring Powers of Attorney must
  - ○ state that the donor has read information to the effect of creating a power.
  - ○ state the donor intends the power to continue in spite of subsequent mental incapacity.
  - ○ state the attorney understands the duty to register in case of the donor's incapacity.
  - ○ be signed by both the attorney and the donor, and the signatures witnessed.
- Registration process
  - ○ Intends to protect against premature use of the power.
  - ○ The attorney must register when the donor is or is becoming incapacitated.
  - ○ 3 relatives of the donor must be notified on registration.
  - ○ Relatives may object to the registration of the power, and the Master of the Court of Protection may decide after holding a hearing.
  - ○ Once registered, there is no routine review to ensure that the donor remains incapable.
  - ○ The Court of Protection may give directions to the attorney regarding the management of the donor's property.
- Practical points
  - ○ Joint attorneys may be appointed – this allows the power to continue on the death of one of the attorneys.
  - ○ The power may range from part to all of the donor's property and affairs.
  - ○ It may take effect immediately or be deferred until the donor becomes mentally incapacitated.
  - ○ The existence of the power does not exclude the donor from making his or her own decisions on those matters in which he or she is capable.
- Proposed reforms to legislation
  - ○ Continuing Powers of Attorney
    - ■ to replace current Enduring Powers of Attorney.
    - ■ allows Attorney to make personal decisions such as health care decisions and consent to medical treatment.
    - ■ a medical certificate of incapacity is necessary for registration.

| Alcohol problems. | *Alcohol misuse*. License revoked until a minimum of 6 months of controlled drinking or abstinence and normalisation of blood parameters. *Alcohol dependency*. License revoked until a minimum of 1 year free from alcohol problems. | *Alcohol misuse*. License revoked until a minimum of 1 year of controlled drinking or abstinence and normalisation of blood parameters. *Alcohol dependency*. License revoked until a minimum of 3 years free from alcohol problems. |
| Drug misuse and dependency. | *Cannabis, amphetamines, ecstasy, LSD.* License revoked until after a minimum 6-month period free of such use. *Narcotics or non-prescribed benzodiazepines.* License revoked until after a minimum 1-year period free of such use. For all types of drug misuse, independent medical assessment and urine screen by DVLA may be required. | *Cannabis, amphetamines, ecstasy, LSD.* License revoked until after a minimum 1-year period free of such use. *Narcotics or non-prescribed benzodiazepines.* License revoked until after a minimum 3-year period free of such use. For all types of drug misuse, independent medical assessment and urine screen by DVLA may be required. |

The effects of psychotropic medication on driving

- No difference whether the drug is prescribed or not.
- All drugs acting on the CNS – may impair concentration, alertness and driving performance. Stop driving if adversely affected.
- Old tricyclic antidepressants – anticholinergic and antihistaminic effects may affect driving performance.
- Newer antidepressants (e.g. SSRI) – generally have fewer adverse effects on driving.
- Antipsychotic drugs – may impair driving performance by their motor or extra-pyramidal effects, sedation and poor concentration.

- Benzodiazepines – most likely to impair driving performance. Alcohol may augment their effects.
- All psychotropic drugs may potentially cause seizures.
- However, patients with mental illness are safer while on regular medication than on irregular or inadequate treatment.

Practical advice for doctors

If a patient has a condition which makes them unfit to drive,

- Make sure that the patient understands that the condition may impair his or her ability to drive.
- If a patient is incapable of understanding this advice (e.g. due to dementia), inform the DVLA immediately.
- Explain to patients that they have a legal duty to inform the medical adviser at DVLA about the condition.
- If the patient refuses to accept the diagnosis or the effect of the condition on their ability to drive, suggest that the patient seeks a second opinion, and make appropriate arrangements for the patient to do so. Advise patient not to drive until the second opinion has been obtained.
- If the patient continues to drive when they are not fit to do so, make every reasonable effort to persuade them to stop (e.g. tell their next of kin).
- If the patient does not stop driving, or if there is evidence that the patient is continuing to drive contrary to advice, consider disclosure of relevant medical information in confidence to the medical adviser at DVLA.
- Before giving information to the medical adviser at DVLA, inform the patient of your decision to do so. Once the medical adviser at DVLA has been informed, write to the patient to confirm that a disclosure has been made.

Human rights legislation

The Human Rights Act 1998

- Came into force on 2 October 2000.
- Incorporates most of the European Convention on Human Rights, which was adopted by most European countries.
- Consists of a set of rights for individuals.

allowed to call witnesses and cross-examine witnesses as in a court of law.

Article 8 – Right to respect for private and family life, home and correspondence
- Breach of confidentiality would not only breach professional code of ethics, it may be a breach of patients' human rights.
- In JT vs United Kingdom (2000), the patient's mother was the designated 'nearest relative' under Mental Health Act 1983 and was entitled to receive confidential information about her daughter. The patient successful argued that as she was unable to change her designated nearest relative, her right for her private life to be respected had been violated.

Mental Health Acts

The Department of Health published a White Paper proposing a new Act to replace the Mental Health Act 1983. At the time of writing, the draft Bill has not passed through parliament. We have given a summary of both the Mental Health Act 1983 and the proposals in the White Paper. However, you must familiarise yourself with the most up-to-date information on this subject, especially if the new Act is passed through parliament.

Key changes in White Paper compared to Mental Health Act 1983

- Broadening of the definition of mental disorder.
- Uniform 3-stage procedures for all patients to replace current section 2/section 3 procedures.
- Compulsory treatment to take place either in hospitals or in the community.
- Distinguishing between patients treated in their best interests and those on the grounds of risks to others in determining care and treatment orders.
- Care and treatment orders to be authorised only by a tribunal chaired by a lawyer in all cases.
- New provisions to detain those with 'dangerous severe personality disorder' who have not committed an offence.

Basic philosophy

Mental Health Act 1983
- Compulsory care and treatment can only be given in hospitals. If patients are not sufficiently ill to require hospital care, they should not lose their civil liberty and autonomy.

White Paper
- Most patients with mentally disorders are now treated in the community. Patients should be provided with treatments in the least invasive and restrictive environment compatible with their safety and welfare.
- Compulsory care and treatment can be given in either community or hospital settings.

Definition of mental disorders

Mental Health Act 1983
- A specific diagnosis is not required under sections 2, 4 or 5.
- For section 3 (compulsory treatment order), the clinician must specify one of the following 4 specific categories of mental disorders
  - Mental illness.
  - Mental impairment.
  - Severe mental impairment.
  - Psychopathic disorder.
- *Mental illness* is not defined in the Act, and is left as a matter of clinical judgement. However, the patient should have one or more of the following features
  - more than a temporary impairment of intellectual functions.
  - more than a temporary alteration of mood so that it gives rise to a delusion or lack of appraisal of his situation.
  - delusional beliefs (persecutory, jealous or grandiose).
  - abnormal perceptions associated with delusional misinterpretation of events.
  - disordered thinking so as to prevent a reasonable appraisal of his situation or reasonable communication with others.
  - mental illness should be of a nature or degree warranting the detention of the patient in the interest of his health or safety.

Place: hospital.
Valid for: 6 months.

a) if the order is primarily for the patient's own interests, the plan must be expected to be of direct therapeutic benefit to the patient.

b) if the order is primarily to protect others from risks, the plan must be considered necessary directly to treat the underlying mental disorder and/or to manage behaviours arising from the disorder.

Place: hospital or community
(but medication will be given against patient's active resistance only in hospitals.
Valid for: 6 months.

Emergency orders

Section 4 (emergency admission to hospital)
Assessed by 1 doctor and an approved social worker.
Criteria
As for section 2, and
- it is of urgent necessity for the patient to be admitted and detained.
- compliance with the usual Section 2 requirements would involve 'undesirable delay'.

Similar to Mental Health Act, except that unlike section 5(2) of MHA 1983, for patients in a hospital other than a specialist mental health unit, recommendations from either 2 doctors or a doctor and a social worker/trained mental health professional are required.

Valid for: 72 hours.
Section 5(2) (for informal
inpatient)
Assessed by 1 doctor.
Valid for: 72 hours.
Section 5(4) (for informal inpatient)
Assessed by 1 registered nurse.
Valid for: 6 hours.
Section 136 (in public place)
Assessed by police.
Valid for: 72 hours.

Patients with long-term mental incapacity

- The House of Lords Bournewood case in 1998 raised the issue about detaining patients incapable of consenting to informal admission (e.g. patients with dementia or learning disability).
- They do not enjoy protection of the safeguards of the mental health act, but there are insufficient resources to invoke the mental health act procedures for all such patients.

The new mental health act provides a new procedure for such patients. The clinical supervisor must

- arrange a full assessment and develop a detailed care plan covering all aspects of care and treatment including any steps which might restrict the patient's freedom.
- arrange an independent doctor to examine the patient. The doctor may suggest changes to the care and treatment plan.
- consult the patient's carers/close relatives and social care representative.
- notify the Commission for Mental Health that a plan is being drawn up.
- finalise the plan within 28 days.
- at any stage, the patient and his or her representative may apply to the Tribunal to challenge or to request a review of the detention. However, it is expected that most cases can be resolved by informal discussion.

Dangerous people with severe personality disorder

- Under the Mental Health Act 1983, dangerous people with severe personality disorders who have not committed an offence and whose conditions are untreatable cannot be detained.

- In the White Paper, the working definition of 'dangerous people with severe personality disorders' is individuals
  - who show significant disorder of personality.
  - who present a significant risk of causing serious physical or psychological harm from which the victim would find it difficult or impossible to recover, e.g. homicide, arson.
  - whose risk appears to be functionally linked to the personality disorder.
- Since one criterion for issuing care and treatment orders is that ''if the order is primarily to protect others from risks, the plan must be considered necessary...to manage behaviours arising from the disorder'', such patients can be detained as long as they pose risks to others, irrespective of the treatability of their conditions.
- This is probably the most controversial part of the White Paper.

2 | Genetics

Chromosomes, cell division, gene structure, transcription and translation

Chromosomes

- Genetic material is stored in pairs of chromosomes in cell nuclei.
- Chromosomes consist of both DNA and its associated proteins.
- In non-dividing cells, chromosomes are uncoiled into threads of chromatin distributed throughout the nucleus.
- In dividing cells, they develop into coiled paired visible structures.
- 23 pairs in humans, 24 pairs in chimpanzees, 39 pairs in dogs.
- *Diploid* – each chromosome is represented twice (one from each parent).
- *Haploid* – each chromosome is represented once (e.g. in reproductive cells).
- *Zygote* – diploid cell formed by union of a male haploid gamete and a female haploid gamete.
- *Sex chromosomes* – the chromosomes which determine the sex of the individual (the 23rd pair in humans, XX for women, XY for men).
- *Autosomes* – chromosomes other than sex chromosomes.

Cell cycle

- Cells alternate between division and non-division.
- Each cycle has 3 phases – interphase, mitosis, cytokinesis.
- Two 46-chromosomal daughter cells result from one 46-chromosomal parental cell.
- Essential for growth and cell replacement.

- Interphase – period of growth and synthesis prior to cell division. 3 stages
  - G1 – rapid growth and synthesis of proteins.
  - S – chromosome and DNA synthesis.
  - G2 – division of mitochondria, formation of spindle fibres.
- Mitosis
  - Interphase – replication of chromosomes.
  - Prophase – condensation of chromosomes, consisting of sister chromatids (identical strand of chromosome) joined at the centre by a single centromere.
  - Metaphase – chromosomes align at the equator.
  - Anaphase – centromeres divide, chromosomes move towards opposite poles.
  - Telophase – chromosomes uncoil.
- Cytokinesis
  - Cleavage at centre of cell, division of cytoplasm.
- Cell division by meiosis
  - Basis of reproduction.
  - Results in the formation of gametes (haploid cell with 23 chromosomes).
  - Diploid ($2n$) cells undergo chromosomal replication once and 2 divisions. Hence, 4 haploid (n) cells are produced.
  - In meiosis I, *paired* homologous chromosomes align at the equator in metaphase I. Hence, 2 diploid cells are produced.
  - In metaphase II, sister chromatids separate in each of the daughter cells to produce 4 haploid cells.
  - Genetic variability of daughter cells are produced by
    - Combination of maternal/paternal chromosomes – in humans, the number of combinations is $2^{23} > 8$ million.
    - 'Crossing-over' – reshuffling of genetic material between sister chromatids in meiosis I.

Gene structure

- A gene is the basic unit of inheritance.
- Genes are part of the chromosome and consist of deoxyribonucleic acid (DNA).
- DNA is made up of 2 strands consisting of nucleotides, running in opposite directions as a double helix.
- Nucleotides are the basic building blocks of both DNA and RNA. Each consists of a base, a phosphate and a sugar.

- DNA bases include adenosine (A), guanine (G), cytosine (C) and thymine (T). In RNA, uracil (U) is used instead of thymine (T).
- Adenosine (A) pairs with thymine (T). Guanine (G) pairs with cytosine (C).
- Genetic information is stored as the sequence of DNA nucleotide bases.
- The information can be decoded as specific proteins to be produced in the cytoplasm. Each 3 consecutive nucleotide bases represent a single amino acid in the protein.
- In addition, it has many non-coding sequences (introns).

Transcription

- A single-stranded messenger RNA is produced from one strand of DNA.
- 3 stages: initiation, elongation and termination.
- *Initiation* – RNA polymerase binds to the promoter region of the DNA. Further unwinding of the DNA occurs.
- *Elongation* – RNA polymerase links RNA nucleotides into a polynucleotide chain. Same base pairing in DNA, except that A (on the DNA) is paired to U (uracil) on the RNA.
- *Termination* – When the RNA polymerase reaches the terminator region, it detaches from the DNA template strand.
- The mRNA is further processed, spliced and moves from the nucleus to the cytoplasm.

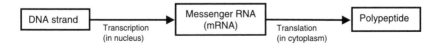

Translation

- The production of polypeptides from the mRNA template.
- Takes place in ribosomes in the cytoplasm.
- Transfer RNA molecules (tRNA) recognise the mRNA triplet nucleotide sequences (codons).
- The other end of the tRNA contains a site that binds to the appropriate amino acid.

○ Associated abnormalities – congenital heart diseases (especially atrio-ventricular canal defects), deafness, cataracts, hypothyroidism, duodenal atresia, Hirschprung disease.
○ Mild to severe intellectual disability.
- Screening
  ○ Age of mother.
  ○ Nuchal translucency.
  ○ Risk increased with elevated human chorionic gonadotrophin (hCG), inhibin A, alpha hCG.
  ○ Risk increased with low α-fetoprotein (AFP), unconjugated estriol and pregnancy-associated plasma protein A.
- Prenatal diagnosis
  ○ Aminocentesis at about 16 weeks.
  ○ Chorionic villus sampling (CVS) at about 10 weeks.

Turner's syndrome (45, XO)

- Short stature.
- Webbing of neck.
- Increased carrying angle.
- Primary amenorrhoea.
- Lack of secondary sexual characteristics.
- Coarctation of the aorta.
- Mild intellectual disability.

Kleinefelter's syndrome (47, XXY)

- Long arms and legs, tall stature.
- Sterility due to low sperm count.
- Gynaecomastia.
- Mild intellectual disability.

Velo-cardio-facial syndrome

- Common chromosomal disorder, about 1 in 4,000 individuals.
- Usually associated with deletions at the long arm of chromosome 22.
- Characteristics
  ○ Variable intellectual disability.
  ○ Cardiac anomalies.
  ○ Pharyngeal hypotonia.
  ○ Cleft palate, abnormal facies.

○ Thymic hypoplasia.

○ Hypocalcaemia due to hypoparathyroidism.

• Abnormal brain imaging in some patients, e.g. reduction in brain volume, reduction of grey matter in various brain regions.

• Behavioural abnormalities

○ Adolescents and children: social withdrawal, abnormal attachment, poor social skills, emotional instability, attention deficits, visuospatial and perceptual deficits.

○ Adulthood: psychotic disorders, especially schizophrenia and bipolar disorders, with prominent auditory hallucinations and exaggeration of pre-existing paranoid traits.

Fragile X syndrome

• Most common inherited disorder, affecting about 1 in 4000 boys and 1 in 6000 girls.

• Caused by the FMR1 gene located on the long arm of the X chromosome.

• When a stretch of DNA in the gene increases beyond a certain length, the gene is switched off and does not produce the normal protein. In carriers, the length is increased but does not exceed this threshold. See dynamic mutation below.

• Males with full mutation have symptoms and signs of the syndrome. Females have milder symptoms as each cell randomly inactivates one of the two X chromosomes.

• Characteristics

○ Long face, large ears and large testes.

○ Intellectual impairment – from mild to severe.

○ Attention deficits.

○ Autistic-like behaviour.

○ Anxiety and unstable mood.

○ Seizures in 25% of cases.

Patterns of inheritance

Mendelian inheritance

Mendel's first law (Principle of Segregation)

During gamete formation, members of a gene pair separate from each other. This explains why the number of genes does not double after each generation.

E.g. when parents with genotypes Rr and Rr are crossed (R stands for dominant allele, r stands for recessive allele)

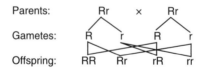

The ratios of RR, Rr and rr are 1:2:1.

Mendel's second law (Principle of Independent Assortment)

During meiosis, genes move randomly and independently into each gamete.

Hence, suppose there are 2 genes, one for eye colour and one for tongue-rolling, whether an offspring inherits the gene for tongue-rolling has no bearing on whether he would also inherit the gene for a particular eye colour.

Single gene characteristics

Terminology

- Genotype – a person's genetic constitution (e.g. sickle cell genes SS, Ss or ss).
- Phenotype – a person's observable properties (e.g. eye colour, symptoms of sickle cell disease).
- Allele – possible alternate forms of a gene (e.g. S or s for sickle cell gene; A, B or O for blood group genes).
- Homozygote – having 2 identical alleles for a given gene (e.g. SS or ss).
- Heterozygote – having 2 different alleles for a given gene (e.g. AO, AB, Ss).
- Dominant – the trait expressed in the heterozygous condition (e.g. since A is dominant over O in blood group, a person with genotype AO has blood group A).
- Recessive – the trait unexpressed in the heterozygous condition (e.g. O is recessive to A in blood grouping).
- Co-dominant – both alleles are fully expressed in the heterozygous condition (e.g. A and B are co-dominant in blood grouping).

- Penetrance – the chance that a person having the diseased genotype will manifest the disease.
- Expressivity – the range of phenotypes resulting from a given genotype.

Autosomal dominant

- Every affected individual usually has an affected parent, except when the individual is a new mutation, or when there is variable penetrance.
- There is a 50% chance of passing on the disease to each child.
- Roughly equal numbers of males and females are affected.
- Children of 2 affected parents have a 1 in 4 chance of being healthy.
- Disease usually less severe than autosomal recessive diseases.
- Examples: Huntington's disease, Marfan syndrome.

Autosomal recessive

- Most affected individuals are children of unaffected parents (usually both parents are heterozygous).
- Children of 2 affected parents are always affected.
- Children of 2 heterozygous parents have a 25% chance of being affected.
- Roughly equal numbers of males and females are affected.
- Disease is usually more severe than autosomal dominant diseases.
- Children of consanguineous marriages are more likely to be affected.
- Examples: most diseases causing enzyme deficiencies, Wilson's disease, cystic fibrosis, phenylketonuria.

Sex-linked recessive

- As X chromosome is much larger than the Y chromosome, most sex-linked conditions are X-linked.
- In X-linked recessive conditions
  - Males are affected much more frequently than females.
  - All daughters of an affected father are carriers.
  - Affected fathers do not pass on the disease to their sons.
  - Half of the sons of heterozygous mothers are affected.
  - Half of the daughters of heterozygous mothers are heterozygous (carriers).
  - Examples include colour blindness, X-linked intellectual disability, haemophilia and muscular dystrophy.

Sex-linked dominant

- There are only a few conditions, e.g. Rett syndrome and hypophosphatemia.
- In X-linked dominant conditions
  ○ Males and females are equally affected.
  ○ All daughters of affected fathers are affected.
  ○ Sons of affected fathers are not affected.
  ○ Half of all children (whether sons or daughters) of affected mothers are affected.

Chromosomal and single gene disorders relating to psychiatry

Single gene disorders			Chromosome disorders	
Autosomal dominant	Autosomal recessive	X-linked disorders (recessive except Rett syndrome)	Autosomal disorders	Sex chromosome disorders
Acute intermittent porphyria	Phenylketonuria	Fragile X	Down's syndrome (trisomy 21)	Turner's syndrome (XO)
Huntington's disease	Wilson's disease	Hunter's syndrome	Edward's syndrome (trisomy 18)	Klinefelter's syndrome (XXY)
Neurofibromatosis	Tay Sach's disorder	Cerebellar ataxia	Patau's syndrome (trisomy 13)	XYY (male, tall, learning difficulties)
Tuberose sclerosis	Hurler's syndrome	Lesch Nyhan	Cri du Chat (deletion 5)	XXX (female, tall, web-necked, learning difficulties)
Von Hippel Lindau		Rett syndrome (X-linked dominant)		

Departure from Mendelian inheritance

Polygenic traits

- Phenotypes that depend on the action of a number of genes.
- These polygenes are also called quantitative trait loci (QTLs).
- The effects of different genes may be additive.
- May result in continuous distribution of phenotypes (e.g. height).

Multi-factorial traits

- Phenotypes that depend on 2 or more genes and a strong interaction with the environment.
- Threshold model – each of a number of genes contribute additively to the genetic liability. Those with a liability above a threshold will develop the genetic disorder if exposed to a certain environmental condition.
- The degree of genetic effects on a trait can be estimated by heritability.

Mitochondrial mutation

- Mitochondria are organelles in cytoplasm that convert energy from carbohydrates to ATP.
- Mitochondria carry DNA molecules responsible for about 37 mitochondrial genes.
- Mitochondria are passed on from one generation to another through the cytoplasm of an egg.
- Hence, diseases due to mitochondrial genes are passed on from the mother, although both males and females can suffer from the disorder.
- Tissues with the highest energy requirements (e.g. nervous tissue, skeletal or heart muscle) are most affected.

Genomic imprinting

- The expression of a gene depends on whether it is inherited from the mother or the father.
- Prader–Willi syndrome
  - characterised by obesity, uncontrolled appetite, intellectual disability.
  - About 60% of cases are associated with a small deletion in the long arm of chromosome 15. Deleted copy is always from the father.
  - About 40% of cases are associated with both copies of chromosome 15 inherited from the mother.
- Angelman syndrome – 'genetic mirror image of Prader–Willi syndrome'

○ characterised by severe intellectual disability, uncontrollable puppet-like movements and outbursts of laughter.
○ About 50% of cases are associated with a small deletion in the long arm of chromosome 15. The deleted copy is always from the mother.
○ About 50% of cases are associated with both copies of chromosome 15 from the father.

Dynamic mutation

- Dynamic changes caused by existence of unstable genomic regions. Examples are trinucleotide repeats and allelic expansion.
- Trinucleotide repeats – mutation associated with an increase in the number of nucleotide triplets in a gene.
- Allelic expansion – increase in gene size due to an increase in the number of trinucleotide sequences.
- Anticipation – more severe symptoms and at earlier ages in successive generations. Initial increase in the number of copies of a trinucleotide repeat causes further progressive increases in successive generations.
- Huntington disease, Fragile X syndrome, Myotonic dystrophy demonstrate these characteristics (trinucleotide repeats, allelic expansion and anticipation).

Genetic epidemiology

Family studies

- Methodology
  ○ Identifies individuals with a given psychiatric disorder (probands).
  ○ Assess their relatives (usually first-degree relatives) for that and other psychiatric disorders.
- Advantages
  ○ Sample collection and assessment are easy.
- Disadvantages
  ○ Can only be used to determine whether a trait is familial, but not whether it is genetic/environmental.
  ○ First degree relatives share similar genetic and environmental factors as the proband.

Twin studies

- Methodology
  - Compare the concordance rates of identical (monozygotic) twins (MZ) with fraternal (dizygotic) (DZ) twins.
  - 2 types of concordance rates: pairwise and probandwise.
  - Pairwise concordance: twin pairs are each counted as one unit. Rate = proportion of pairs in study sample in which both twins have the disorder.
  - Probandwise concordance: each affected twin is a unit of analysis. Rate = proportion of affected twins whose co-twins also have the disorder.
  - Probandwise is often slightly higher than pairwise concordance.
  - Concordance rate can be interpreted as an intraclass correlation.
  - If concordance rates are high for both MZ and DZ, suggests strong environmental influence.
  - If concordance rates $MZ \gg DZ$, suggest strong genetic influence.
- Advantages
  - Easy to recruit patients.
- Disadvantages
  - Bias may occur as twins may believe they are special and behave differently.
  - MZ twins may share more environmental factors than DZ twins.

Adoption studies

- Methodology
  - Compare rates of psychiatric morbidity
    a. adoptee studies – adoptees whose biological parents have the affected disorder vs control adoptees.
    b. adoptee's family studies – adopted individuals with the disorder are ascertained. Studies the rates of disorder amongst their biological vs adopted relatives.
    c. Cross-fostering studies – adoptees with affected biological parents and unaffected adoptive parents vs those with unaffected biological parents and affected adoptive parents.
  - If relative risk high for both adoptees and adoptive parents, suggest environmental influence.
  - If association between adoptees and biological parents high, suggest genetic influence.
- Assumption: adoptees are randomly placed with adoptive parents.

Combination designs

- Combine twin and family studies (e.g. compare twin with siblings)
  - Need to adjust for age differences.
  - Generally, findings from combination designs give hereditary/ environmental effects more similar to those from twin studies than adoption studies.
- Combine twin and adoption studies
  - Recruitment difficult: very few twins are now reared apart.

Molecular genetic designs

Rely on DNA markers to locate a gene without knowing how the gene works.

Allelic association

- The correlation between a DNA marker and a measured characteristic is calculated for a population.
- A correlation implies that the gene influences the trait.
- Useful in detecting continuous distributed traits multi-factorial in origin.
- Advantages
  - Easy to recruit subjects.
  - Allows use of existing data-sets, easy to repeat analysis.
- Disadvantages
  - False positives due to population stratification – variation in genetic-make up in a population may not be due to the trait under study.

Linkage analysis

- Study of the correlation between the extent to which family members share a given DNA marker and their similarity for a given disorder.
- Since genes located close together are more likely to be inherited together (without crossover), a correlation implies that the gene influences the disorder.

Molecular genetic techniques

DNA polymorphisms

- These are genetic sites with frequent DNA sequence variations (over 2% of the population).

- They are of no clinical consequences if they occur
  - in non-coding DNA.
  - in coding DNA but do not result in changes in amino acids.
- Useful as markers for studying the inheritance of both normal and abnormal genes.
- 2 broad types:
  - *Site polymorphism* – DNA point variations (i.e. restriction fragment length polymorphism, RFLP).
  - *Length polymorphism* (e.g. variable number of tandem repeats).

Restriction enzymes

- Enzymes which cut DNA only at specific sequences.
- Found naturally in bacteria.
- So far, about 500 restriction enzymes have been identified with over 100 different recognition sites for DNA cleavage.

Gene probes

- Sections of single-stranded DNA labelled with radioactive or non-radioactive substances.
- If they are mixed with single-stranded DNA made up of sequences complementary to the probe, a labelled double-stranded molecule will be formed and can be visualised.
- Hence, specific gene probes are useful for identifying specific DNA sequences.

Restriction fragment length polymorphism

- Restriction enzyme = cutting enzymes (enzymes which cut DNA fragments).
- Slight but unique differences in the banding pattern of DNA fragments from different individuals are revealed when subjected to restriction enzyme analysis. These variations in the DNA are called restriction fragment length polymorphisms (RFLPs).
- Therefore useful as a marker in genetic linkage maps.

Schizophrenia

- Mean concordance rates MZ pairs = 46%, DZ pairs = 14%.
- Afro-Caribbeans living in UK have higher incidence than those living in West Indies, suggesting environmental risk.
- Overall, suggest gene–environmental interaction.
- A gene named 'disrupted in schizophrenia (DISC1)' may be important for cortical development and schizophrenia pathogenesis.
- Other possible candidate genes include neuregulin-1 and dysbindin.

Autism

- Both family studies and twin studies suggest a strong genetic influence.
- Concordance rates MZ 75% vs DZ 4%.
- Substantial increase in social deficits in relatives of autistic patients.
- Much genetic heterogeneity – some have no demonstrable genetic abnormalities, others do (e.g. fragile X syndrome in 5%, tuberose sclerosis in 3%).

Drug and alcohol problems

- Family studies – alcohol and drug problems tend to run in families and genetic factors play a substantial role.
- Molecular genetic studies – Asians have lower rates of alcoholism due to flushing response from a variant of the ALDH2 gene.
- Drug use – genetic and environmental factors seem to be equally important.

Prenatal identification and genetic counselling

Value of prenatal identification

- Discuss options if diagnosis confirmed (e.g. abortion).
- Reassurance for parents if no disease is found.
- Prepare parents practically and psychologically for the birth of an affected child.
- Arrange appropriate services for the early management of the child.
- Reassess chance of disorder in next pregnancy and discuss options.

Genetic counselling

Includes

- Consultation with family and arranging investigations.
- For each family member, give
  - information about condition.
  - risk of developing the condition.
  - risk of transmitting the condition.
- Non-directive in order to help families choose options appropriate for their needs.

Organisation of clinical genetic services

- Currently regional genetic centres offer specialist services to families at high risk of serious genetic disorders.
- Services provided include: diagnosis, risk estimation, counselling, surveillance and support.
- The centres are multi-disciplinary, with
  - Clinical staff – medical geneticists and counsellors (who may have backgrounds in nursing or social work).
  - Laboratory staff – molecular genetics (DNA analysis) and cytogenetics (chromosome analysis).
- Referrals may be made by primary care or hospitals.
- E.g. children with a learning disability may be referred by paediatricians after they have excluded non-genetic causes.

DNA banks

- Collection of human genetic material, either through routine sampling or for specific purposes.
- Examples include
  - collection of neonatal blood sample for Guthrie test.
  - from volunteers in a certain age band (e.g. Biobank UK project).
- Purposes at a population level
  - to study the epidemiology of genetic alleles.
  - elucidate genetic-environment interaction at a population level.

3 | Epidemiology

What is epidemiology?

- It is the study of disease in populations.
- Time, place and person
  - Time – when people get diseases, variation with season, changes of disease occurrence over time.
  - Place – where they are when they get diseases, geographical variation (locally, regionally, nationally, or internationally).
  - Person – who is affected, e.g. in terms of their age, sex, occupation, socioeconomic group, etc.
- Results are useful for
  - devising strategies to prevent the disease.
  - planning services for the management of the disease.
  - monitoring the level of disease, as a time trend and to compare between different geographical areas.
  - exploring new treatment methods if the aetiology is better known.

Basic concepts and measures in epidemiology

Measuring diseases

- Define 'case' – several possible methods
  - *Statistical* – e.g. 2 standard deviations from the mean.
  - *Clinical* – e.g. threshold level of symptoms or signs.
  - *Prognostic* – e.g. alcohol consumption above which risks to health increase significantly.
  - *Operational* – may be pragmatic based on level of treatment.

- Population
  - *Study population* – we must specify explicitly in which population we are measuring diseases (e.g. all men between 50 and 65 on 1 January 2003 living in the Eastern Region of England).
  - *Population at risk* – the population at risk includes those in the study population who might develop a disease. For example, only women who have not had a hysterectomy are at risk of cancer of the uterus.
- Study sample
  - Usually, we do not have the information on everyone in the study population. So, we select a few (i.e. our study sample).
  - To ensure that the disease rates in our sample reflect our study population, we must use a valid sampling method (see below).
- Measuring disease frequency

  Incidence
  - The rate at which new cases occur within a given period of time.
  - = number of new cases/(population at risk × time period).
  - E.g. in a school with 1,000 pupils, there were 5 new cases of meningitis in the 6-month period between 1/1/2003 and 1/7/2003).

  Incidence = $5/(1,000 \times 0.5) = 1$ per 100 person-years at risk.

  Prevalence
  - *Point prevalence* – the proportion of a population who have the disease at any one point in time.
  - *Period prevalence* – the proportion of a population who have the disease at any time within a given period.
  - Point prevalence is usually lower than period prevalence. Point prevalence is not suitable for acute diseases.
  - E.g. in a school with 1,000 pupils, there are 70 pupils suffering from asthma.

  Prevalence = $(70/1,000) \times 100\% = 7\%$.

  Risk
  - The chance of any one person developing a disease within a given period of time.
  - = number of new cases/population at risk during the period.
  - In a school of 1,000 pupils, 400 pupils were immune to chickenpox. 5 pupils develop chickenpox between 1 July 2003 and 1 January 2004. What is the risk of developing chickenpox in the 6-month period?

  Population at risk = $1,000 - 400 = 600$.

  Risk = $(5/600) \times 100\% = 8.3\%$.

Age groups	Number in study groups	Prevalence of death from disease in reference group	Expected cases
<44	500	1%	5
45–64	1,000	2%	20
>65	500	4%	20
			Total = 45

Hence, the study population has a lower death rate than expected. Standardised mortality rate $= 20/45 = 44.4\%$.

Measures of association between cases, disease and exposure surveys

Comparing disease rates in exposed vs unexposed groups

- Simply comparing incidence of disease amongst groups in the population exposed and unexposed to certain risk factors (e.g. men with women, smokers vs non-smokers, asbestos workers vs other workers).
- Must ensure the same standard disease definition (e.g. ICD classification) is used in both groups.
- *Attributable risk* = risk in exposed persons − risk in unexposed persons.
- *Relative risk* = risk in exposed persons/risk in unexposed persons.
- *Population attributable risk*
  = absolute number of diseases avoided if the factor is eliminated.
  = attributable risk × prevalence of disease.
- ***Attributable proportions*** = proportion of disease which would be eliminated in a population if disease rate is reduced to those in unexposed persons.
- Main disadvantage is the risk of confounding variables distorting results (see below).
- Age and sex as confounders can be minimised using direct or indirect standardisation techniques.

Case-control studies

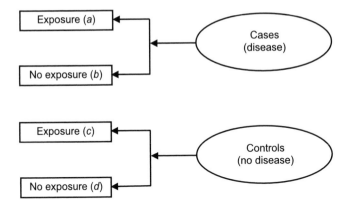

- A group of patients with the disease is compared to another group without the disease. Their previous exposures to the factor in the two groups are also compared.
- Identify cases
  - need robust case definition.
  - new (i.e. incident) case identification usually better than prevalent cases.
- Identify controls
  - exposure level must be similar to the general population.
  - free of the disease or symptoms.
  - matched to each case (e.g. in age, sex).
  - exposure levels must be possible to measure.
  - 2 common sources: general population (e.g. general practice registers) or similar patients with other diseases.
- Calculation of association
  - Odds ratio $= ad/bc$.
  - Odds ratio $> 1 \rightarrow$ exposure associated with disease.
  - Odds ratio $< 1 \rightarrow$ exposure protects against disease.

Cohort studies

A group of people sharing a certain experience at a point in time is followed up for a period of time to determine whether they develop an outcome of interest, e.g. a disease. Most cohort studies are prospective.

- *Identify a cohort* – must be unambiguously defined, i.e. all people in a certain town or all people exposed to a certain trauma (e.g. in the study of post-traumatic stress syndrome).
- Define risk factors to be studied and the outcome to be followed up.
- Record baseline information – all likely relevant factors for the development of the disease under study should be recorded.
- Follow-up the cohort – keeping track of subjects can be difficult (e.g. due to change of address).
- Calculate association – relative risk (RR) $= \dfrac{b(a+b)}{d(c+d)}$.

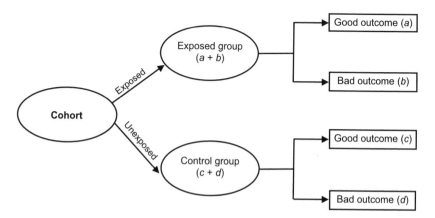

Comparison of case-control and cohort studies

		Type of study	
		Case-control study (Retrospective)	Cohort study (Usually prospective)
Advantages of case-control over cohort study	Time to perform	Quick	Takes time
	Resources	Cheap	Expensive
	For rare diseases	Appropriate approach	Large sample needed
	Drop-out	Not a problem	Considerable problem

Advantages of cohort over case-control study	Selection of cases and controls	Considerable problem	Not relevant
	Recall bias Incidence of disease	Considerable problem Does not give incidence of disease	Not relevant Gives incidence of disease
	Results	Odds ratio	Relative risk

Both methods may be biased due to confounding variables.

Sources of epidemiological data

Relevant sources include the following
- Population
  - Census data – populations nationally, within a district, or by age/sex/socio-economic status or ethnic group.
- Mortality
  - National registration of deaths and their causes (via death certificates).
- Morbidity
  - National and local registers – e.g. cancer registers, congenital abnormalities.
  - Communicable disease notifications.
  - Morbidity data from General Practice national studies.
  - Prescribing data.
- Health care
  - Hospital returns to Department of Health – e.g. numbers of finished consultant episodes, number of discharges and deaths.
  - Hospital Episode Statistics (HES) – based on individual records. Includes diagnosis, length of stay, and clinical data.
  - Health service indicators.

Methods of sampling

- Purpose of sampling
  - inadequate time and resources to collect data on every subject in our study population.

- o to ensure that the sample is representative of the subjects in our study population, so that we can generalise our results from the sample to the population.
- Methods
  - o Simple random sampling
    - ▪ Draw up a sampling frame – a list of subjects in the study population.
    - ▪ Generate random numbers to select subjects.
  - o Systematic sampling
    - ▪ Draw up a sampling frame.
    - ▪ Select every nth subject on the sampling frame (assume $1/n$ of the population were to be selected).
    - ▪ Advantage: quick and convenient.
    - ▪ Disadvantage: possible bias if there is an association between the ordering in the sampling frame and the factor being studied.
  - o Multi-stage random sampling
    - ▪ E.g. to sample 1,000 secondary school students in UK, we can first randomly sample 10 schools and then randomly sample 100 students from each school.
    - ▪ More practical and convenient.
  - o Stratified random sampling
    - ▪ A method to ensure that the distribution of a factor (e.g. age, sex) in our sample is the same as the population.
    - ▪ Divide the population into different strata. Take random samples from each stratum.

How to interpret associations

Association

- E.g. subjects exposed to a risk factor (e.g. alcohol) are more likely to have certain diseases (e.g. cirrhosis, suicide).
- Indicated by a relative risk >1 in cohort studies OR odds ratio >1 in case-control studies.
- Association does **not** necessarily mean the risk factor causes the disease.

Possible explanations for association

- *Chance finding.* Type I error – if we regard $p < 0.05$ as statistically significant, we will find a positive association in 1 out of 20 studies even if there were no actual relationship between the risk factor and the disease.
- *Spurious finding.* There may be methodological weaknesses causing systematic bias. E.g. sampling bias, recall bias in case-control studies.
- *Confounding factors.* The association may be due to a third factor positively associated with the putative risk factor and disease. E.g. we may find that heavy smokers are more likely to have liver cancer. However, this may be because people who are heavy smokers are more likely to be heavy drinkers as well, and heavy drinking is related to liver cancer.

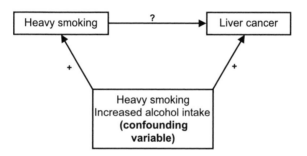

- *Reverse causation.* For example, the association between low social class and schizophrenia does not necessarily mean that low social class causes schizophrenia. An alternative explanation is that patients suffering from schizophrenia are more likely to drift down the social class ladder.

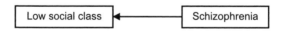

- *Causation.* The risk factor causes the disease.

Criteria that support an association being causal

If there is an association between a risk factor and a disease, the following criteria tend to support (though not prove) the hypothesis that the risk factor causes the disease.

- *Consistency.* Studies carried out in different populations at different times by different researchers arrive at the same conclusions
- *Biological plausibility.* There is a biological explanation why the risk factor might cause the disease.
- *Strength of association.* Very high relative risk or odds ratio, i.e. subjects exposed to the risk factor are *much* more likely than non-exposed subjects to have the disease.
- *Dose response relationship.* i.e. The greater exposure to the risk factor, the more likely it is to have the disease.
- *Temporal relationship.* The disease develops *after* exposure to the risk factor.
- *Reversibility.* If the risk factor is removed (e.g. smoking cessation), the probability of developing the disease decreases.
- *Specificity.* The putative risk factor is associated with only one disease and no other. However, this rarely occurs in real life.

Explanations for variation in morbidity

Differences in levels of morbidity
- Levels of morbidity differ depending on many factors, e.g. age, sex, ethnicity, social class.
- Generally, morbidity increases with age.
- Women consult doctors more often than men, but women live longer.
- People in lower social classes (e.g. class V) generally have the highest morbidity.

Triangular causation of disease. The presence of disease is caused by the interaction of 3 factors:

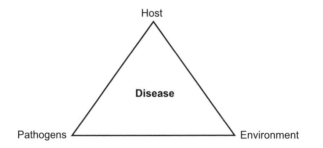

- The host – its genetics, physiology, social environment, habits (smoking), etc.
- The pathogen – e.g. infective agents.
- The environment – e.g. social overcrowding, asbestos.

The web of causation. The factors contributing to diseases are complex. They include the following categories.

- Physiological and clinical – including genetic components and current physiological factors (e.g. body mass index).
- Behavioural – e.g. alcohol and drug misuse, smoking.
- Social, environmental and political – e.g. work or unemployment, social class, social isolation, stress.

These factors help to explain variations in morbidity.

The iceberg principle of care

- Out of all those with a disease, only a small proportion are symptomatic.
- Of all those with symptomatic diseases, only a few are aware of them.
- Out of all those who are aware of their symptoms, only a small proportion seek the advice of health professionals.
- Out of all those seeking advice, only a proportion are seen by health professionals.
- Out of all those seen by health professionals, only a proportion are appropriately treated and helped.

Stages on the pathway to care in psychiatry

General population ⇔ develop psychiatric symptoms → consult general practitioner → symptoms correctly detected by general practitioner → referral to psychiatrist.

Factors determining whether a mental disorder is detected

Patient factors

- How it is presented (e.g. somatic presentation more difficult to detect).
- Severity of disorder (i.e. mild symptoms are more easily overlooked).
- Previous history of psychiatric problems.
- Frequency of recent consultations (i.e. chance of detection increases with frequency).

Doctor factors

- Attitude to mental disorder.
- Knowledge and interest in psychiatry.
- Assessment bias (e.g. ethnic minority may be more likely to be misdiagnosed).
- Skills in mental state examination.
- Empathy and use of non-verbal cues.

Screening

- Use of a simple test to detect a disease before it presents itself.
- E.g. screening for alcohol misuse amongst GP patients, routine recording of blood pressure.

Wilson's criteria on the usefulness of a screening test

- The condition should be an important health problem.
- An acceptable form of treatment or useful intervention (e.g. genetic counselling) exists for patients with the recognisable disease.
- The natural history of the condition should be reasonably well understood.
- A recognisable latent or early symptomatic stage exists.
- The test for detecting the disease at an early or latent stage is
  - simple and acceptable to patients.
  - accurate (i.e. high sensitivity and specificity).
- Facilities are available for the diagnosis and treatment of the patients uncovered during screening.
- An agreed policy exists on whom to treat.
- The treatment at the pre-symptomatic stage of the disease should favourably influence its course and prognosis.
- The programme is cost-effective.

Measurement of accuracy of screening tests

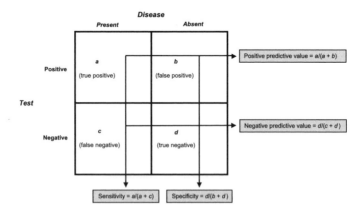

Explanation of terms

Terms	Definition	Changes when prevalence increases	Applicable to a population with different prevalence of disease?
Sensitivity	Amongst subjects with disease, the proportion correctly diagnosed by test	Constant	Yes
Specificity	Amongst subjects without disease, the proportion correctly excluded by the test	Constant	Yes
Positive predictive value	For a subject tested positive, the probability that the subject has the disease	Increases	No
Negative predictive value	For a subject tested negative, the probability that the subject is disease free	Decreases	No

Estimating needs, concept of supply and demand

Need, demand and supply

- Need – interventions with capacity to benefit.
- Demand – what the patients asked for.
- Supply – health care actually provided.

		• Appropriate for sensitive topics (e.g. HIV)
Disadvantages	• People's reasons for their views or feelings cannot be explored • Interviewees can only give a minimal response • Designing questionnaires requires much expertise	• Requires good interviewing skills • More interviewees are needed to make general comparisons • As the questions are not prescriptive, thoroughly planned preparation is essential • Analysis of the data may require more skills • Takes more time and resources
Analysis	Often statistical	Often combining statistical with qualitative analysis

4 | Principles of evaluation and psychometrics

Types of data

Dependent and independent variables

○ In research, we often try to make predictions of some variables given our knowledge of other variables. E.g. prediction of treatment outcomes from the age, sex, ethnicity, diagnosis and other factors.
○ Dependent (outcome) variables – the variables we are trying to predict.
○ Independent (predictive or explanatory) variables – the variables which we have information about.

Types of scales

1. **Nominal (categorical) scale.** Observations are put into categories but not graded. Examples include eye colour, nationality, gender and blood group. If there are only 2 categories, they are also known as a *binary* or *dichotomous* scale. Examples include gender, answers to a yes/no question and home ownership.
2. **Ordinal (ranked) scale.** Observations are put in *categories* which are graded (i.e. ranked). However, the differences between any two categories are not necessarily the same or even measurable. An example is social class. One cannot assume the difference between social classes I and II is the same as the difference between social classes IV and V.

    Other examples include examination grades (e.g. A, B, C, etc.), council tax banding and Likert scale in a questionnaire (e.g. strongly agree, agree, neutral, disagree, strongly disagree).

Note that most scales used in psychiatry (e.g. anxiety or depression scales) are ordinal scales although the measurements are given a numerical scale. For example, the difference between a Beck's depression scale of 20 and 24 is not necessarily the same as that between 24 and 28.

3. Interval scale. On this scale, differences between 2 observations are measurable and meaningful. However, there might not be a meaningful 'zero point', and the ratio of 2 observations might not be meaningful.

For example, temperature measurements in Fahrenheit or Centigrade are interval scales but not ratio scales. The difference between, say, $20°C$ and $30°C$ is the same as the difference between $30°C$ and $40°C$. However, one cannot say that $20°C$ is twice as hot as $10°C$. (The 'true zero' is actually $-273°C$.)

4. Ratio scale. Ratio scale is a special type of interval scale for which there is a meaningful 'zero point', and the ratio of 2 observations is meaningful. Examples include weight, height, plasma cholesterol level and blood pressure.

Different designs for studies

There are 3 basic designs for studies

- Independent groups design
  - Characteristics of 2 or more groups of subjects are compared.
  - E.g. responses to treatment between male and female groups, or between different age-groups.
  - Usually, the mean or variance of the observations of one group is compared to another.
  - Unpaired statistical tests (e.g. independent t-test) are usually appropriate.
- Repeated measures design
  - Repeated observations are made of the same subjects.
  - E.g. blood pressure is taken of the same subjects before and after an experimental treatment.
  - Paired statistical tests (e.g. paired t-test) are usually appropriate.
- Matched subjects design
  - A group of subjects with a pre-defined characteristic (i.e. the 'cases') is identified.
  - For each 'case', a predetermined number (often 1) of control subjects similar to the case apart from the characteristic being studied are identified. This forms the matched control group.

○ The aim is to compare the outcomes of the cases and controls.
○ The case-control study is one example of matched-subject designs.

Common research study types

■ Cross-sectional studies – see below.
■ Case-control studies – see epidemiology section.
■ Cohort studies – see epidemiology section.
■ Randomised controlled trials – see below.

Cross-sectional studies (or prevalence studies)

• Aim to measure 'how common' (the prevalence) a disease, risk factor (e.g. smoking, alcohol intake), or view (e.g. health belief) are in a defined population.
• Sampling of a group of people representative of the defined population at a particular point in time.
• Caution required to interpret relationship between variables, as confounding may occur.
• Steps:
  1) Sampling. Random sampling to ensure that the subjects selected are representative of the population under study (see types of sampling in epidemiology section).
  2) Obtaining data. There are 3 important steps:
     a) Deciding what to collect – there are 2 main sets of data to collect:
        • Dependent variables: the outcome data.
        • Independent variables: characteristics which may influence the outcome data (e.g. age, sex, social class).
     b) Deciding how to collect the data
        • E.g. postal questionnaires, interviews, or from existing documents.
        • Data must be collected in a standard manner (e.g. using a standard questionnaire or interview proforma).
     c) Securing a satisfactory response rate
        • E.g. ensuring adequate explanation to subjects and reminders to non-responders.
        • A satisfactory response rate is important, as non-respondents may differ significantly from responders in the outcome measures.
        • The impact of non-response to the validity of the study can be assessed by comparing these characteristics with those of the responders. If the profiles of non-responders differ significantly from responders, the results of the study should be treated with caution.

Prediction and hypotheses

Basic steps

An important aim of research is to draw conclusions. We do this by setting up a hypothesis and testing it. The basic steps are as follows:

1. *State the 'neutral' position (i.e. null hypothesis).* The null hypothesis is usually the position we want to disprove – e.g. there is no difference in the characteristics between 2 subject groups. The alternative hypothesis (e.g. there is a difference between the 2 groups) is the one we want to prove.
2. Find the probability (p value) that the value of the test statistic has occurred by chance (i.e. if the null hypothesis were true).
   a) Determine the appropriate statistical test. The appropriate test depends on several factors:
      - the types of variables (e.g. categorical, ordinal, interval).
      - whether the variables are normally distributed.
      - whether we are comparing means or proportions.
      - whether data is paired or not.
      - what the null hypothesis is.
   (See later in this chapter)
   b) Calculate the test statistic.
   c) Look up the p value in relevant statistical tables.
3. Decide whether the probability is so small that the null hypothesis is so unlikely that it can be rejected
   - $p < 0.05$ means that the probability of obtaining the test statistic if the null hypothesis were true is less than 1 in 20.
   - $p < 0.05$ is traditionally used as a cut-off point to conclude that the null hypothesis (that there is no difference) is too unlikely to be true.
   - $p > 0.05$ means that the probability of obtaining the test statistic if the null hypothesis were true is over 1 in 20 – i.e. it is not very unlikely. In other words, we have not shown one way or another whether there is a difference.
4. *Draw the relevant conclusions*
   - If $p < 0.05$, the null hypothesis is very unlikely and therefore the alternative hypothesis is true (i.e. there is a significant difference between 2 groups).
   - If $p > 0.05$, the null hypothesis is not so unlikely that it can be dismissed (i.e. we have not shown one way or the other whether a difference exists).

Although $p = 0.05$ is often used as a threshold, different p values have been used to show how strong the evidence is. A more practical way of interpreting p value is

p value	Strength of evidence of a relationship or difference
<0.001	Very strong
<0.01	Strong
0.01–0.05	Some
0.05–0.1	Doubtful
>0.1	Little or none

1-tailed and 2-tailed tests

E.g. we wish to show that drug A gives better outcome than placebo. The null hypothesis for a:

- 2-tailed test – the outcomes of both drug A and placebo are identical. The alternative hypothesis is either that drug A is better than placebo or that drug A is worse than placebo.
- 1-tailed test – drug A is worse than or equal to placebo. The alternative hypothesis is that drug A is better than placebo.

1-tailed tests usually give a smaller (i.e. more highly significant) p value than the corresponding 2-tailed test. 2-tailed tests are almost the norm in clinical research. 1-tailed tests should only be used on rare occasions when it is impossible for an effect to be in one direction.

Confidence intervals

- 95% confidence intervals of the differences between the 2 groups are often more useful to indicate how precise our results are.
- The strict definition is the range of the differences found on 95% of the occasions if the study were carried out many times.
- They are often loosely interpreted to mean the values between which the real difference lies with a probability of 95%.

For example, we may wish to compare the mean systolic blood pressure between 2 groups of patients. If the difference is reported as 10 (95% CI 4 to 15), we know the likely difference in blood pressure lies between 4 and

15 mmHg. Since the interval does not include zero, we can also conclude that the result is significant at $p < 0.05$ level.

Conversely, if the difference is 5 (95% CI − 5 to 10), we know that although the estimated difference is 5 mmHg, it can lie between − 5 and 10. In other words, the difference could be zero. This corresponds with the result that it is not significant at $p < 0.05$ level. We can also conclude that even if there is a difference, it is unlikely to exceed 10 mmHg.

Type 1 and type 2 errors

Type I error (α):

- The test detects a difference when there is no actual difference.
- Type I error rate is the same as the p value.

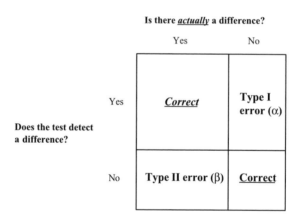

Type II error (β)

- The test fails to detect a difference although there is actually one.
- Type II error rate is equal to 1 − power (e.g. a test with a power of 80% has got a type II error rate of 20%).

Power

- Power – the probability that a test will produce a significant difference at a given significance level (e.g. $p < 0.05$) if there is a given true difference between the 2 populations compared.

- Power $= 1 - \beta$, where β is the type II error rate.
- Power increases if
  1. the variation (e.g. standard deviation) of the variables is smaller,
  2. the actual differences between the 2 populations are larger,
  3. the sample size is larger,
  4. the significance level is lower (i.e. higher p value).

Sample size calculation

In conducting research, we ask a different question: what is the minimum sample size needed to detect a given difference between the 2 populations at a certain significance level with a certain probability? (i.e. How many subjects are needed to detect a difference of 15 mmHg in blood pressure between the 2 groups at $p < 0.05$ with a power of 80%?)

The sample size increases (i.e. we need more subjects) if:

- the difference we wish to detect is less.
- the variation (e.g. standard deviation) of the variable increases.
- the level of significance increases (i.e. p value is smaller).
- the power required increases.

Controlling for confounding variables

- Apart from randomised controlled trials, all the above research designs are liable to misleading results caused by confounding variables.
- If the confounding variables are unknown, they cannot be controlled for.
- For known potential confounding variables, they may be controlled for by
  - Stratification
    - A simple method.
    - E.g. if sex is a potential confounding variable, the results may be analysed separately for male and female subjects.
  - Regression analysis
    - A useful method for controlling for several potential confounding variables.
    - Independent variables: the treatment group the subject is randomised to, all potential confounding variables.
    - Dependent variable: the outcome variable of the study.

Clinical trials

Basic schema of randomised controlled trials

- An experiment to evaluate
  - the effectiveness of an intervention (e.g. treatment, preventive measures) by comparing the outcomes of a group receiving intervention with a control group (i.e. who receive either placebo or traditional intervention) OR
  - the aetiology of a disease by exposing one group of subjects to one set of factors and the *other* group to another set of factors.
- Main advantage: minimise risk of bias due to known or unknown confounding variables.
- Steps
  1. Defining a study population.
  2. Determine number of patients required.
  3. Determine eligibility criteria. Unambiguous justifiable criteria are necessary.
  4. Randomisation into treatment and control groups
     Aim to ensure that baseline characteristics of the 2 groups are similar. In randomisation, each subject has a pre-determined chance of being allocated to each group, but the group to be allocated cannot be predicted. Concealment – allocation to treatment arms must be concealed from patient and clinician. Otherwise, this may influence the clinician's decision to recruit patients or the patient's consent to the trial.

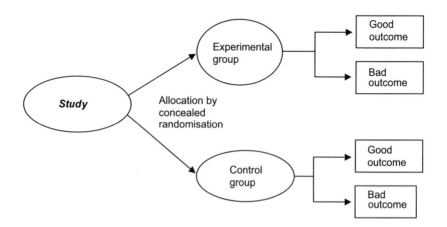

Criteria for concealment
- The person who generates the allocation sequence should not be the person who determines eligibility and entry of patients.
- Treatment allocation should be decided by people not involved in the trial.

Types of randomisation
- *Simple randomisation* – e.g. use of sealed envelopes, random number generated by computer, etc.
- *Block randomisation* – e.g. a block of 3 may mean randomly assigning subjects in 3s according to the regime (ABC, ACB, BAC, BCA, CAB, CBA). The aim is to ensure similar numbers of patients are allocated to each group.
- *Stratified randomisation* – to ensure the groups are balanced for certain prognostic factors which are known to be related to outcome.

5. Intervention – use of placebo control. It may be impractical or unethical to use placebo in the non-intervention group:
- for treatments other than drugs.
- if an existing treatment has been shown to be more effective than placebo
  - Double blind – both the subjects and the clinicians do not know the treatment allocated.
  - Single blind – the subjects do not know what treatments they are receiving, but the clinicians do.
  - Purpose of blinding – to minimise placebo effects (for patients) and differences in clinicians' enthusiasm in delivering treatment.

6. Assessment of outcome – at the beginning of the trial, the following details on the outcome should be determined:
- The outcomes are clinical measurements, death, length and/or quality of life, etc.
- Outcomes may be primary or secondary.
- Blinding in assessment – both patients and investigator should be blind to the outcome.

7. Analysis according to 'intention to treat' (or worst-case scenarios)
- Intention to treat analysis – for patients who
  - drop out of the study or
  - are non-compliant with the treatment assigned

should be analysed according to the group to which they were originally allocated. This method maintains the advantages of random allocation.
- Worst case scenarios – assuming drop-outs who were originally allocated to the 'treatment' group had the worst possible outcomes,

Trials with small and large sample sizes

- *n-of-1 trials*
  - One subject receives the experimental intervention at one time and the control at a different time.
  - The results only apply to 1 patient and cannot be generalised.
  - Useful for rare diseases for which no evidence is available.
- *A mega trial*
  - A clinical trial using simple designs involving collection of a large number of patients across multiple centres.
  - The aim is to increase sample size and hence statistical power of the trial.

Trials with and without pre-determined numbers of subjects

- *Sequential trials*
  - Parallel trials in which the number of subjects is not pre-determined by the researchers beforehand.
  - Subjects are recruited until a clear conclusion (i.e. the intervention is useful or harmful or no significant difference) is reached.
  - Advantage: Maximise efficiency by avoiding either unnecessarily excessive number of subjects or too few subjects.
  - Disadvantage: The outcome must be measurable soon after the trial begins.
- *Fixed size trials*
  - The researcher determines the sample size before the trial starts.
  - The number is decided either by sample size calculation or pragmatically.
  - Advantage: Useful if the outcomes cannot be determined until some time after the trial begins
  - Disadvantage: Risk of recruiting too many or too few subjects, as the assumptions of sample size calculations may not be correct.

Preference trials

- In simple RCTs, patient's preference determines whether they consent to participate in a trial.
- This may bias the results if their preference is related to the outcomes.
- 3 trials attempt to address this by taking into account patient's preference

Zelen's design

■ Subjects are randomised before they give consent to take part in a trial.
■ Those who are randomised to standard treatment are told they are not part of a trial.
■ Those who are randomised to experimental treatment are given a choice to participate or not.
■ Those who refuse are given standard treatment but are analysed within the experimental group.
■ Advantage: All eligible subjects are included and selection bias due to patient preference minimised.
■ Disadvantages: Blinding not possible. Power of trial may be reduced by a large proportion of refusal to participate. Ethical concern of monitoring those who refuse participation.

Preference trial with comprehensive cohort design

■ All subjects are followed up irrespective of whether they were randomised.
■ Those who refused to participate in the trial are given the interventions they prefer, and followed up as if they were part of a cohort study.
■ The object of the trial is to compare those in the RCT and those in the cohort studies.
■ Useful if a large proportion of subjects are likely to refuse to participate.

Wennberg's design

■ Patients are randomised into 'preference group' and 'RCT group'.
■ Those in the 'RCT' group are randomised to receive different interventions.
■ Those in the 'preference group' are given the treatment the subjects prefer.
■ The impact of patient's preference is analysed by comparing the RCT group and the preference group.

Descriptive statistics

Frequency and probability distributions

Frequency distributions
■ *Frequency* – The number of observations having a particular value.
■ *Frequency distribution*

Definitions

Variance $= s^2 =$ sums of squares/degrees of freedom $= \Sigma(x_i - x)^2/(n-1)$, where n is the number of observations and x is the mean of all observations. An easier way to calculate variance is variance $= [\Sigma x_i^2 - (\Sigma x_i)^2/n]/(n-1)$. *Standard deviation* $= s = \sqrt{Variance}$.

Quartiles. Quartiles are values dividing the data set into parts so that there are equal numbers of observations in each part. For example, the upper quartile is the value which a quarter of all observations lie above it. The lower quartile is the value which a quarter of all observations lie below it. Similar definitions can be given to deciles (i.e dividing the data set into 10 parts) and centiles (i.e. into 100 parts). The interquartile range is the difference between the upper and lower quartiles.

Range. The range is the interval between the highest and lowest value. Sometimes, it is defined as the difference between the highest and the lowest value.

Graphical representation of the distribution of a variable

The appropriate graphical representation to describe the frequency distribution of the data depends on the types of data.

Types of data	Nominal or ordinal	Continuous data (interval or ratio)
Types of chart	Pie chart Bar chart	• Histogram (for discrete data, e.g. number of children, age band) • Frequency distribution curve • Box and whisker plots • Cumulative frequency curve

Box and whisker plot

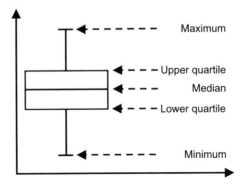

Skew data

For continuous data, data are skewed if the distance from the central value to the extreme is much greater on one side than the other.

Positive skew (i.e. skewed to the right) – Tail on the right longer than tail on the left, mean > median.
Negative skew (i.e. skewed to the left) – Tail on the left longer than tail on the right, median > mean.

Specific parametric and non-parametric tests for group comparison

Parametric tests

Parametric tests assume that the data are on an interval scale and normally distributed. They generally have a higher power than non-parametric tests, especially when the sample size is small.

a) Comparing means of 2 large samples

When the sample size is large, the sample means are normally distributed irrespective of the distribution of the observations (Central Limit

We can then calculate the *p* value (with the null hypothesis that their mean is zero) and their 95% confidence interval using the *t* distribution. The assumption is that the variable is normally distributed in the population.

However, if the sample size is large, the normal distribution can be used (Central Limit Theorem) even if the distribution of the variable is skewed.

Non-parametric tests

These tests do not assume the data are distributed according to certain families of distributions (e.g. normal distribution). Generally, they are based on the rank order of data and can be used for ordinal variables. Their main disadvantage is that they have less power than their corresponding parametric tests especially when the sample size is small.

a) The Mann–Whitney U test

This is the non-parametric equivalent of the independent sample *t*-test. The null hypothesis is that subjects in one group do not exceed the other group overall. To perform the test, arrange all the observations in the 2 groups in ascending order. Rank orders are assigned to all observations, and the value *U* is calculated from the rank orders of the members of each group. The relevant *p* value can be looked up in a statistical table.

b) Wilcoxon matched pair test

This is the non-parametric equivalent of the paired *t*-test. It is applied to paired data and the null hypothesis is that there is no tendency for one set of data to be higher or lower than the data paired to. The data must be on an interval scale. First, the absolute differences between the paired data (i.e. ignoring the positive and negative signs) are calculated and assigned a ranked order. Second, the sum of the rank orders for the positive differences and negative differences are calculated. Finally, these are compared and assessed for statistical significance.

c) Sign test

Like the Wilcoxon matched pair test, this is a non-parametric test for paired data. However, it can be used for ordinal data as the test only considers whether the data in one group is larger or smaller than its matched data in the other group. It has less power than the Wilcoxon matched paired test.

Statistical tests for comparing groups

	Parametric tests		Rank order tests	
	Test	Assumption	Test	Assumption
Comparing means or medians of 2 groups	Normal test Independent sample *t*-test	Large sample Variable normally distributed with uniform variance in the 2 groups	Mann–Whitney *U* test	
Comparing 3 or more groups	1-way analysis of variance (*F* test)	Variable normally distributed Homoscedasticity (i.e. uniformity of variance)	Kruskal–Wallis analysis of variance	Homoscedasticity
Paired comparison (e.g. before and after)	Normal distribution Paired *t*-test	Large samples Variables normally distributed	Wilcoxon matched pair test Sign test (can be used for ordinal data)	Interval scale

Relationship between 2 variables

Regression is a technique to investigate how well 1 variable can be predicted from 1 or more other variables. It can be used to:

- investigate the relationship between 2 or more variables, with or without adjusting for confounding variables.
- predict one variable from other variables.

For example, one might be interested to know how well smoking habit and social class predict the incidence of lung cancer. It is important to identify the following types of variables in a regression analysis:

If the independent variable is an interval variable, the adjusted odds ratio is the factor by which the odds must be multiplied for a unit increase in the independent variable.

Situation	Types of regression
One predictor (independent) variable, interval outcome (dependent) variable	Simple linear regression
2 or more predictor (independent) variables, interval outcome (dependent) variable	Multiple regression
Binary outcome (dependent) variable	Logistic regression

Reliability and validity

Indices of effectiveness of a measuring instrument

Reliability

- The repeatability of the instrument in measuring the same phenomenon.
- 3 aspects of reliability: agreement, stability and internal consistency.
- *Agreement aspects* – e.g. inter-rater reliability (i.e. agreement between 2 observers) and parallel form agreement (i.e. agreement between 2 forms of the same test to the same group of people). Measured by intraclass correlation coefficient (ICC).
- *Stability aspects* – e.g. test–retest reliability (i.e. same group of people taking the same test 2 or more times).
- *Internal consistency* – one single measurement instrument is administered to one group of subjects at one time. The reliability of the instrument is determined by the correlation of the items that reflect the same constructs. Measured by Cronbach's Alpha.

Intraclass correlation coefficient (ICC)

- An estimate of inter-rater reliability.
- Calculated from estimates of within-subject variance (s_w^2) and between-subject variance (s_b^2) by

$$ICC = \frac{s_b^2}{(s_b^2 + s_w^2)}.$$

- ICC varies from 0 (no agreement) to 1 (perfect agreement).

Cronbach's Alpha

- An index of internal consistency of the results of a rating scale or questionnaire.
- Between 0 and 1. A higher score indicates higher level of internal consistency.
- Scores of 0.7–0.8 are generally regarded as satisfactory.

Validity

- Are the results from our measuring instruments true?
- Components of validity: face validity, content validity, criterion validity (including predictive and concurrent validity) and construct validity.
- *Face validity* – its relevance for the purpose of the study or the subjects we wish to measure.
- *Content validity* – its relevance to both the purpose of the study and to experts in the field.
- *Criterion validity* – the ability of the instrument to predict or agree with constructs external to that we are measuring. Includes
  - *Predictive validity* – ability to predict external constructs. E.g. can an IQ test predict the future academic success of a child?
  - *Concurrent validity* – ability to give results consistent with other co-existing constructs. E.g. do the results of an IQ test agree with the opinion of the children's teachers?
- *Construct validity* – the ability of the instrument to produce results in agreement with other related constructs in the expected manner. E.g. do the results of a depression score agree with those of anxiety rating scales or other depression rating scales?

Analysis	Grounded theory approach, constant comparative method	Statistical
Data for reporting	Highlighted quotes from subjects	Statistical results
Reasoning	Inductive (from specific to general)	Deductive (from general to specific)
Strength	Validity	Reliability

Participant observation

- Observing behaviour in a real-life setting while taking a role in the setting at the same time.
- Involves a balance of being a participant (i.e. subjective immersion) and a researcher (i.e. being scientific, neutral and objective).
- Items of observation
  - The setting.
  - The participants and communication patterns.
  - Activities and behaviour – including inactivities.
  - Informal activities and communication.
  - Verbal and non-verbal language.
  - Documents – e.g. memoranda, mission statements, minutes of meetings.
- Record as field notes.
- Variation of participant observations
  - Role of observers – may be partial or full participants.
  - Portrayal of role to others – range from full disclosure to all participants to disclosure to only some participants (e.g. only managers).
  - Portrayal of study purpose to others.
  - Duration of observations – range from 1 hour to several years.
  - Focus of observation – range from a single element to broad focus.
- Advantages
  - Naturalistic situation and credible.
  - Less risk of Hawthorne effects.

Discourse analysis

- Detailed study of naturally occurring talk.
- Has origins from linguistics, sociology and psychology.

- Analysis of how small elements in talk contribute to a set of discourses which actively construct a specific way of looking at the world.
- Examples of types of discourses for doctors:
  - personal experience discourse (i.e. connected with personal feelings),
  - professional discourse (i.e. relating to a doctor's professional practice),
  - institutional discourse (i.e. how doctors frame their professional practice experience into discourses appropriate for the institution, as in a departmental meeting).
- Also analyses how such discourses might confer authority or 'power' on the speaker.
- The elements analysed include: tone, pauses, interruptions, non-verbal communications, words used and their connotations, turn-taking.
- Usually involve analysis of transcripts of natural talk.
- May be used to study why a doctor's style is authoritative, patients' unspoken messages and why certain discourses are perceived as 'correct'.

Single case studies

- Usually involves study of a single subject, but may also include study of a single system (e.g. family or couple).
- Usually involves the study of the effects of an intervention (e.g. drug treatment, psychotherapy, educational or social intervention, etc.) on a well-defined outcome (e.g. Beck depression score).

Single case study research designs

- ABA design (Classic reversal)
  - A – baseline data is recorded.
    B – intervention introduced.
    A – intervention stops.
  - If treatment is effective, there will be an improvement in phase B but returns to baseline when treatment stops.
- Other variations
  - ABAB design – provides more support if there is improvement when the second period of intervention starts (see the Figure below).
  - ABAC design – useful for testing more than one intervention.

5 | Neuroscience

Neuroanatomy

Organisation of the nervous system

Central nervous system (CNS)
- Consists of brain and spinal cord.
- Acts as the control centre of the body.

Peripheral nervous system (PNS) – consists of neurones connecting the CNS with muscles, receptors and glands. Divided into:
- Afferent system – neurones carry information from periphery to the CNS.
- Efferent system – neurones carry information from CNS to the periphery. Subdivided into:
  - Somatic nervous system (SNS) with efferent neurones carrying impulses from CNS to skeletal muscle. Under conscious control = voluntary.
  - Autonomic nervous system (ANS) with efferents from CNS to smooth muscle, cardiac muscle and glands. Not under conscious control = involuntary system. 2 divisions of ANS:
    - Sympathetic.
    - Parasympathetic.

Meninges

Meninges are coverings around the brain and spinal cord. Consist of 3 layers:

- Dura mater
  - Outer layer of dense fibrous connective tissue.
  - Epidural space between dura mater and bone.

- Arachnoid mater
  - Thin connective tissue membrane.
  - Subdural space between dura and arachnoid mater.
- Pia mater
  - Transparent fibrous membrane.
  - Innermost layer closest to neural tissue.
  - Subarachnoid space between pia and arachnoid mater, cerebrospinal fluid (CSF) circulates in this space.

Ventricular system

Ventricles are fluid-filled cavities in the brain. Contain choroid plexus, a vascular tissue that secretes cerebrospinal fluid.

- Lateral ventricles
  - found in each hemisphere of cerebrum under corpus callosum.
  - extend into frontal, occipital and temporal lobes.
  - drain through interventricular foramina into third ventricle.
- Third ventricle
  - vertical slit between and inferior to the thalamus, between lateral ventricles.
- Fourth ventricle
  - between inferior brainstem and cerebellum.
  - connected to the third ventricle by the cerebral aqueduct.

Cerebrospinal fluid (CSF):

- CSF is a clear watery liquid containing glucose, urea, salts, some lymphocytes and a small amount of protein.
- Made by filtration and secretion from capillaries in the ventricular choroid plexus.
- Circulates through lateral, third and fourth ventricles before entering subarachnoid space.
- Reabsorbed into veins at a rate equal to the rate of production.

Functions:

- Protection of nervous tissue.
- Delivers nutrients and removes waste.

Blood supply to the brain

Blood reaches the brain through the vertebral arteries and internal carotid arteries.

- Frontal eye field
  - Involved with conjugate eye movements and voluntary scanning of the eyes.
- Broca's area
  - Located on the inferior frontal gyrus.
  - In the dominant hemisphere – left for most people.
  - Involved in the motor part of speech.
  - Sends messages to the premotor area that co-ordinates speech muscles.
  - Damage causes expressive dysphasia.
- Prefrontal cortex
  - Involved in aspects of personality, initiative, judgement and depth of feeling.
2. Parietal lobe – lies behind central sulcus, lateral fissure forms ventral boundary, parietooccipital sulcus forms posterior boundary. Important areas include:
   - Primary somaesthetic (somatosensory) area
     - Located on the postcentral gyrus.
     - Receives sensations from receptors in various parts of the body.
     - Mapped to form a sensory homunculus.
     - Localises exact point from which sensations originate.
   - Secondary somaesthetic area
     - Located in dorsal wall of lateral sulcus and may extend onto the insula.
     - Involved in less discriminative sensation.
   - Somaesthetic association area
     - Located in the superior parietal lobule on lateral surface of the hemisphere.
     - Integrates and interprets sensations.
     - Stores memories of previous sensory experiences.
     - Inputs received from the thalamus and primary somaesthetic area.
   - Angular and supramarginal gyri.
     - Involved in perception and interpretation of spoken and written language.
3. Temporal lobe – important areas include:
   - Primary auditory area
     - Located on the superior temporal gyrus.
     - Interprets basic characteristics of sound.
   - Secondary auditory area (auditory association area).
     - Lies behind the primary auditory area.

- Interprets sounds and associates auditory inputs with other sensory inputs.
- Wernicke's area
  - Sensory speech area.
  - Dominant hemisphere.
  - Connected to Broca's area by the arcuate fasciculus.
  - Interprets the meaning of speech. Damage causes receptive dysphasia.
- Primary and secondary olfactory areas.
  - Interprets sensations relating to smell.
- Hippocampus.
  - Inputs from neocortex, parahippocampal gyrus and entorhinal cortex.
  - Main outputs to entorhinal cortex and ventral striatum.
  - Close links to septal nuclei through the fornix and fimbria.
  - Fornix allows information to travel between hippocampus and the hypothalamus, septum, thalamus and midbrain.
- Entorhinal cortex
  - Anterior part of parahippocampal gyrus.
  - Included in the lateral olfactory area.
- Parahippocampal gyrus.
  - Lies next to hippocampus, part of hippocampal formation.
  - Receives sensory information from association areas.
- Amygdala.
  - Located in medial temporal lobe.
  - Pathways – stria terminalis and ventral amygdalofugal.
  - Connects to hippocampus via entorhinal cortex.
  - Also connects to hypothalamus and sensory cortical areas.
4. Occipital lobe – anterior border formed by parietooccipital sulcus. Important areas include:
   - Primary visual area.
     - Located on the medial surface and may extend on to the lateral surface.
     - Interprets shape, colour and movement.
   - Visual association area.
     - Receives information from the primary visual area and the thalamus.
     - Identifies and recognises visual responses.

Basal ganglia

The basal ganglia are paired masses of grey matter in each cerebral hemisphere. They are made up of:

Hypothalamus

Group of nuclei at base of the brain below thalamus and just above pituitary. Forms floor and part of the lateral walls of the third ventricle. Divided into different regions:

- Supraoptic
  - Contains paraventricular nucleus, supraoptic nucleus, anterior hypothalamic nucleus, suprachiasmatic nucleus.
- Tuberal region
  - Contains hypophyseal tract that transports hormones into blood vessels. Ventromedial, dorsomedial and arcuate nuclei.
- Mammillary
  - Contains mammillary bodies and posterior hypothalamic nucleus.
  - Fibres of the fornix mainly end here.

Functions:

- Control of hunger, thirst, and body temperature.
- Involved in primitive emotional reactions, e.g. rage and aggression.
- Links endocrine and nervous systems, e.g. controls pituitary.
- Acts as pacemaker to drive many biological rhythms, e.g. waking and sleep patterns.
- Controls and integrates autonomic nervous system, e.g. regulates heart rate, smooth muscle and secretion from glands.
- Receives and integrates sensory input from viscera.

Epithalamus

Contains pineal gland and structures involved in autonomic responses to emotional changes.

Subthalamus

Contains subthalamic nuclei and neuronal tracts passing to the thalamus. Parts of the reticular formation, the red nucleus and substantia nigra may extend into the subthalamus.

Limbic system

Ring of structures connected together. Functional system rather than anatomical. Composition of the limbic system varies between textbooks.

The limbic system may consist of the following structures:

- Cingulate gyrus.
- Subcallosal gyrus.
- Hippocampal formation (dentate gyrus, hippocampus, subiculum, part of parahippocampal gyrus).
- Primary olfactory cortex.
- Septal area.
- Amygdala.
- Hypothalamus (mammillary body).
- Thalamus (anterior and dorsal nuclei).

These structures are connected by:

- Fornix.
- Papez circuit.
- Stria terminalis.
- Medial forebrain bundle.

Receives inputs from all sensory systems and the neocortex. Outputs via amygdala and hypothalamus.
Functions of the limbic system:

- Emotional and behavioural responses.
- Memory.
- Survival instincts.

Brainstem

Forms the stalk from which the cerebral hemispheres and cerebellum sprout. Relays information between the cerebrum, cerebellum and spinal cord. Medial lemniscus is a band of white fibres passing through the brainstem; it carries information about fine touch, proprioception, pressure and vibration sense to the thalamus. Provides the face and neck with sensory and motor functions via the cranial nerves. Regulates vital functions, e.g. breathing, consciousness. Divide into the medulla, pons and midbrain.

Medulla

- Direct continuation of the spinal cord.
- Extends from foramen magnum of skull to the inferior part of the pons.
- Contains nuclei and white matter.

- White matter contains all the ascending and descending tracts between the spinal cord and brain.
- Motor tracts are located in the pyramids and most fibres decussate to the opposite side of the body just above the junction of the medulla and spinal cord.

Nuclei include:

- Cranial nerve nuclei VIII, IX, X, XI, XII.
- Nucleus gracilis and nucleus cuneatus receive sensory fibres from ascending tracts and relay sensory information to the opposite side of medulla.
- Olivary nuclei send projections to the cerebellum to control movement.
- Vestibular nuclei help to control sense of equilibrium.
- Reticular formation.
- Reflex centres to control heart rate, breathing and blood vessel diameter.

Functions

- Conduction pathway for motor and sensory information.
- Consciousness and arousal from sleep.
- Controls cardiovascular and respiratory systems.
- Co-ordinates swallowing, vomiting, coughing.

Pons

Lies above medulla and anterior to the cerebellum.
Contains:

- White matter:
  - Longitudinal fibres – motor and sensory tracts.
  - Transverse fibres – pass to cerebellum through middle cerebellar peduncles.
- Nuclei of cranial nerves V, VI, VII, VIII (vestibular).
- Reticular formation – area to control respiration.

Midbrain

Extends from pons to lower part of diencephalon.
Contains:

- Fibre bundles called cerebral peduncles that contain some motor and sensory fibres. Main connection for tracts between upper part of brain and lower parts of brain and SC.
- Substantia nigra – large pigmented nucleus near cerebral peduncles.

- Cranial nerve nuclei III, IV.
- Superior colliculi – centres for reflexes involving head, neck and eye movements with visual and other stimuli.
- Inferior colliculi – centres for reflexes involving head and body movements with auditory stimuli.
- Midbrain reticular formation. Red nucleus of reticular formation receives fibres from cerebellum and cerebrum. Origin of rubrospinal tract.

Cerebellum

Located at the back of the brain behind the cerebrum. Consists of 2 lateral hemispheres separated by the vermis. High number of neurones – >50% of the total in the CNS. Sits on peduncles – bundles of fibres arising from the brainstem:

- Inferior peduncles receive spinocerebellar tracts and input from the vestibular nuclei of the medulla. Connect cerebellum with medulla. Afferent and efferent fibres.
- Middle cerebellar peduncles only receive signals from cerebrum via tracts that synapse in the pons. Connect cerebellum with pons.
- Superior cerebellar peduncle fibres leave cerebellum and travel to midbrain. Mostly efferent information.

Functions:

Role in controlling movement:
  - Co-ordinate subconscious skeletal muscle movements.
  - Maintain equilibrium and control posture.
  - Process information to produce smooth co-ordinated movements.
  - Predict future position of body parts during movement.
Deep cerebellar nuclei relay cerebellar information to parts of the brainstem involved in descending spinal pathways.
May help modulate emotions.

Anatomy of cranial nerves

The cranial nerves carry information from the special senses and somatosensory receptors to the brain. Supply skeletal muscles in head and parts of trunk. Provide parasympathetic innervation to smooth muscles and glands in the head and thorax. Neurons begin or end on clusters of neurones within the brainstem called the cranial nerve nuclei.

- *Olfactory nerve (I):* Arises in olfactory mucosa, passes through cribriform plate to the olfactory bulb. Olfactory tract arises from the bulb and ends in the primary olfactory areas of cortex.
- *Optic nerve (II):* Arises in retina of eye, passes through optic foramen and forms the optic chiasma. Optic tracts pass through the lateral geniculate nucleus in the thalamus and end in visual areas of cortex.
- *Oculomotor nerve (III):* Motor division arises in midbrain, passes through supraorbital fissure to muscles of upper eyelid and eyeball for movement of eyelid and eyeball. Provides parasympathetic innervation to the ciliary muscle and iris to produce accommodation and pupil constriction. Sensory fibres from eyeball muscles pass to midbrain to allow proprioception.
- *Trochlear nerve (IV):* Motor division arises in midbrain, passes through superior orbital fissure to superior oblique extra-ocular muscle. Sensory fibres from this muscle pass to midbrain to allow proprioception.
- *Trigeminal nerve (V):* Motor division arises in the pons and ends in muscles of mastication to enable chewing. Sensory fibres come from 3 divisions and end in pons:
  Ophthalmic – sensation from upper face and forehead.
  Maxillary – sensation from mucosa of nose, palate, upper jaw.
  Mandibular – sensation from anterior 2/3 of tongue, lower teeth and skin over mandible and cheek.
- *Abducens nerve (VI):* Motor division arises in pons, passes through superior orbital fissure to lateral rectus extra-ocular muscle. Sensory fibres from proprioceptors in this muscle pass to pons.
- *Facial nerve (VII):* Motor division arises in pons, passes to muscles of face, scalp and neck. Provides parasympathetic supply to lacrimal and salivary glands. Sensory fibres from anterior 2/3 of tongue pass through geniculate ganglion in pons, then through the thalamus to gustatory areas of cortex.
- *Vestibulocochlear nerve (VIII):* Cochlear branch arises in spiral organ of ear, forms spiral ganglion, passes through medullary nuclei to thalamus, synapse with neurones going to auditory areas of cortex. Vestibular branch arises in semi-circular canal, saccule and utricle, forms vestibular ganglion and ends in thalamus.
- *Glossopharyngeal nerve (IX):* Motor division arises in medulla passes to parotid gland for salivary secretion. Sensory fibres from posterior 1/3 of tongue and carotid sinus pass to thalamus for control of swallowing, taste and regulation of blood pressure.
- *Vagus nerve (X):* Motor division from medulla to respiratory passages, heart, smooth muscle and glands of upper GIT. Sensory fibres from these organs pass to medulla and pons.

- *Accessory nerve (XI):* Motor division arises in medulla passes to muscles of pharynx, larynx and soft palate to control swallowing. Spinal division to neck/shoulder muscles for head movement. Sensory fibres from muscles carry proprioceptive information.
- *Hypoglossal nerve (XII):* Motor division arises in medulla passes to tongue muscle for movement, speech and swallowing. Sensory fibres from tongue to medulla for proprioception.

Anatomy of spinal cord

Begins at the foramen magnum at the base of the skull and ends opposite the disc between L1 and L2. Covered by same meninges as the brain. Contains:

- Grey matter core
  - Forms the anterior and posterior horns.
  - Cell bodies are grouped into clusters of nuclei (laminae).
  - Amount varies depending on volume of tissue supplied by spinal nerves at that level, e.g. more where neurones leave to supply the limbs.
- White matter
  - Surrounds grey matter.
  - Consists of longitudinal running fibres of the ascending and descending tracts. Selected tracts are shown on the following diagrammatic representation:

Cross-section of the spinal cord:

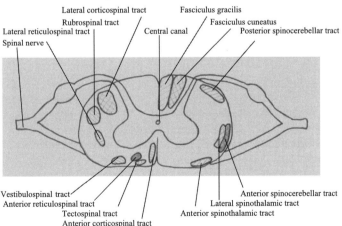

Cross-section of the SC

Ascending pathways

Fasciculus gracilis and fasciculus cuneatus:

- Fasciculus gracilis carries information from lower body, fasciculus cuneatus carries information from upper body.
- Axons enter dorsal column, ascend SC and synapse in the dorsal column nuclei of the medulla.
- Decussate in the medulla, called internal arcuate fibres.
- Axons then form the medial lemniscus, relay in ventral posterior nucleus of the thalamus and pass to the somatosensory cortex.
- Carries sensory information of discriminatory touch, proprioception and vibration.

Spinocerebellar tract:

- Originates in posterior grey horn, ascend in the lateral column and synapse in the cerebellum.
- Carries subconscious proprioceptive information.
- Anterior and posterior tracts – posterior tract carries ipsilateral information, anterior tract carries bilateral information.

Lateral spinothalamic tract:

- Fibres synapse in dorsal horn, and after entering SC decussate in anterior white commissure.
- Ascend SC in lateral column to the ventral posterior nucleus of thalamus.
- Fibres join medial lemniscus and pass to the somatosensory cortex.
- Carries pain and temperature sensation.

Anterior spinothalamic tract:

- Fibres synapse in dorsal horn and decussate in anterior white commissure.
- Ascends SC in the anterior column to the ventral posterior nucleus of the thalamus.
- Fibres join medial lemniscus and pass to the somatosensory cortex.
- Carries touch and pressure sensation.

Descending pathways

Lateral corticospinal:

- Originates in motor cortex, descends through corona radiata and internal capsule.
- Tracts decussate in the medulla and descend in the lateral column to synapse in the anterior grey horn.
- Carries motor impulses that co-ordinate precise discrete movements.

Anterior (ventral) corticospinal:

- Originates in motor cortex, descends ipsilaterally in anterior column to the anterior grey horn. Fibres may cross in SC.
- Carries motor impulses that co-ordinate the axial skeleton.

Rubrospinal:

- Originates in midbrain, descussates, descends in the lateral column to the anterior grey horn.
- Carries motor impulses that co-ordinate precise discrete movements.

Reticulospinal:

- Lateral tract originates in medulla and descends in the lateral column. Carries motor impulses that inhibit extensor reflexes and muscle tone.
- Anterior tract originates in pons and descends in the anterior column. Carries motor impulses that facilitate extensor reflexes and muscle tone.

Vestibulospinal:

- Originates in medulla, descend in anterior column.
- Carries motor impulses to maintain body tone in response to head movements.

Tectospinal:

- Originates in midbrain, descend in anterior column.
- Carries motor impulses to control head in response to auditory, visual and cutaneous stimuli.

Types of cell found in the nervous system

There are 2 main categories of cells in the nervous system – neurones and neuroglia:

- Neurones receive and transmit information by the release of neuro-transmitters at synapses.
- Neuroglia are cells that support neuronal function by providing support, nourishment and insulation.

Neurones

Considerable variation in size and shape. Typical neurone consists of:

Neuronal membrane

- 5 nm thick phospholipid bilayer.
- Protein pores and pumps cross the membrane.
- Keeps neuronal cytoplasm together and prevents some extracellular substances from entering the cell.

Cell body (soma or perikaryon)

- Contains the nucleus and cytoplasm.
- The nucleus is surrounded by a double membrane (nuclear envelope) and contains chromosomes and messenger RNA.
- Cytoplasm is made up of a potassium rich solution (cytosol), rough and smooth endoplasmic reticulum, mitochondria and Golgi apparatus.

Cytoskeleton

- Microtubules, microfilaments and neurofilaments maintain the shape of the neurone.

Dendrites

- Processes that branch out from the cell body and may form a dendritic tree.
- Covered in synapses. Some have dendritic spines that may isolate specific chemical reactions and receive only some types of synaptic input.

Axon

- Arises from the axon hillock where it leaves the cell body.
- Length varies from <1 mm to >1 metre, they often branch.
- Diameter varies from <1 to 25 micrometres. Electrical signals propagate faster with greater axon diameter.
- The terminal bouton is at the end of the axon where it contacts other cells and passes on electrical signals.

Synapse

- Specialised junctions that enable communication between neurones.
- Presynaptic membrane forms a swelling (bouton).
- Presynaptic terminal contains synaptic vesicles and mitochondria.
- Postsynaptic membrane shows thickenings.
- Pre and postsynaptic membranes are separated by the synaptic cleft – a gap of about 20 nm.

Neuroglia in the central nervous system

Astrocytes

- Star shaped multi-polar cells with several thick processes.
- Commonest type of neuroglia, provide structural support for neurones.
- Form the blood–brain barrier and enable the passage of nutrients and metabolites between the neurones and the blood.
- Regulate the chemical content of the extracellular space.
- Regulate neurotransmitters by restricting their spread and removing them from the synaptic cleft.
- Role in scar tissue formation.

Oligodendrocytes

- Smaller cell body and fewer processes.
- Main function is to lay down myelin to form the myelin sheathes of the neurones in the CNS. One oligodendrocyte may myelinate several different axons. These sheathes have gaps (nodes of Ranvier) where the neuronal membrane is exposed. These help to speed neural transmission.

Microglia

- Small, thin, elongated cells.
- Found throughout CNS but particularly prevalent in grey matter.
- Respond to damage to the CNS.
- Act as scavengers and use phagocytosis to remove debri, e.g. dead neurones, glia.

Ependymal cells

- Ciliated cells that form the epithelial lining of cavities in the CNS and assist movement of the cerebrospinal fluid (CSF).
- Role during brain development to direct cell migration.

- 3 types:
  - Ependymocytes – line ventricles and central canal of the spinal cord.
  - Tanycytes – line floor of the third ventricle and have processes next to capillaries to actively transport metabolites from the blood into CSF.
  - Choroidal epithelial cells – form epithelium of the choroidal plexuses and secrete CSF.

Neuroglia in the peripheral nervous system

Schwann cells

- Provide layer of membrane insulating axons.
- One cell myelinates a single axon.
- Support neurones, produce and maintain myelin.
- Role in regeneration of peripheral nerves.

Major white matter pathways

White matter consists of the myelinated axons of neurones. There are 3 different types of fibres:

1. Association fibres – connect neurones between gyri in the same hemisphere, e.g. superior longitudinal fasciculus, arcuate fasciculus.
2. Commissural fibres – connect corresponding areas of the 2 hemispheres, e.g. corpus callosum, anterior and posterior commissures.
3. Projection fibres – connect the cerebral cortex and subcortical structures, brainstem and spinal cord, e.g. internal capsule, ascending and descending tracts.

Corpus callosum

- Connects the 2 cerebral hemispheres.
- Fibres from an area of cortex in one hemisphere end in corresponding area in the other hemisphere.
- Lies above diencephalon at the inferior end of the longitudinal fissure.

Fornix

- Made of fibres forming the major output pathway from the hippocampus.
- Connects hippocampal formation of each temporal lobe with the hypothalamus (especially mammillary bodies).
- Involved in limbic system.

Papez circuit

- Ring of interconnected neurones
- Impulses travel in both directions around the circuit.
- Part of the limbic system.
- Inputs from neocortex, thalamus, septal area, raphe nuclei, ventral tegmental area, and reticular formation.
- Output to neocortex and reticular formation.
- Forms link between limbic system and neocortex.
- Complete circuit: hippocampus (via fornix) to mammillary bodies – thalamus – cingulate gyrus – hippocampus.
- Role in emotion, perception, memory and certain types of behaviour.

Other circuits relevant to integrated behaviour

See section on integrated behaviours in neurophysiology.

Major neurochemical pathways

Dopaminergic pathways

Nigrostriatal

- Arise from cells in the substantia nigra and pass to the putamen.
- Involved in extrapyramidal disorders.
- Concerned with sensorimotor co-ordination.
- Damage causes Parkinsonism.

Mesolimbic

- Arise in ventral tegmental area and pass to many components of the limbic system including the hypothalamus and hippocampal formation.
- May be involved in the positive symptoms of schizophrenia.
- Some drugs used to treat schizophrenia block action of this pathway.
- Associated with noradrenergic innervation of the limbic system.

Mesocortical

- Arise in ventral tegmental area and pass to the neocortex especially prefrontal areas.
- May be involved in the negative symptoms of schizophrenia.

Ascending noradrenergic pathways

Locus coeruleus in the pons gives rise to ascending efferent fibres.
2 pathways:

1. Dorsal tegmental bundle
   o Ascends in midbrain and becomes part of the medial forebrain bundle when reaches the hypothalamus.
   o Fibres sent to forebrain structures via forebrain bundle, cingulum, stria medullaris and the fornix.
   o Midbrain branches to periaqueductal grey matter, tectum, dorsal raphe nucleus, geniculate nuclei and other lateral thalamic nuclei.
   o Telencephalon branches to amygdala, hippocampal formation, septal area, olfactory centres and entire neocortex.
2. Dorsal periventricular pathway
   o Enters periaqueductal grey of midbrain and innervates parts of the hypothalamus.

Pathways have roles in

- Fear, anxiety and stress dampening.
- Sleep, attention focussing and vigilance.
- Neurodegenerative diseases, depression and schizophrenia.

Cholinergic pathways

Basal forebrain cholinergic pathway

- Fibres originating in septal nuclei
  o Project to habenula and base of midbrain.
  o Some fibres travel in fornix to hippocampus and dentate gyrus.
  o Other fibres to hypothalamus and olfactory bulb.
- Fibres originating in basal nucleus of Meynert project to cerebral cortex and amygdala.
- Receives inputs from:
  o Cortical areas – orbitofrontal, entorhinal, temporal.
  o Subcortical areas – septal nuclei, nucleus accumbens and hypothalamus.
- Role in memory, affective behaviour and complex behaviours dependent on emotional and motivational states.

Brainstem cholinergic pathway

- Cholinergic neurones found in reticular nuclei in brainstem.
- Fibres form lateral and medial tegmental columns.
- Dorsal tegmental cholinergic pathway passes to midbrain tectum, geniculate bodies and thalamus.
- Ventral tegmental cholinergic pathway passes to thalamus and hypothalamus.
- Role in arousal and sleep.

Serotonergic (5-HT) pathways

Serotonergic neurones are located in brainstem raphe nuclei. Descending, intrinsic brainstem, cerebellar and ascending projections:

- Descending bundles end in dorsal and ventral grey columns of the spinal cord, run length of cord and influence cell columns.
- Intrinsic brainstem projections arise from pontine and midbrain serotonergic neurones and synapse on cells of the locus coeruleus, tegmental nuclei and reticular formation.
- Cerebellar projections arise from pontine cell groups and pass to cells of cerebellar cortex.
- Ascending fibres form dorsal and ventral bundles.
  - Dorsal ascending serotonergic bundle arises from pontine cells and ends in midbrain reticular nuclei, periaqueductal grey and parts of hypothalamus.
  - Ventral ascending serotonergic bundle forms part of central tegmental fasciculus of midbrain and supplies substantia nigra, thalamus, lateral hypothalamus, mammillary body, striatum and limbic system, hippocampus via fornix and cingulum, amygdala, septal areas, entorhinal cortex and olfactory areas.

Role in:

- Pain control.
- Sleep.
- Depression.
- Facilitation of spinal motor neurones, sympathetic control, inhibition of catecholinergic neurones.

Glossary

Afferent – heading towards centre.
Claustrum – thin layer of grey matter between insula and lentiform nucleus.

Contralateral – on the opposite side.

Decussation – crossing over.

Efferent – going away from centre.

Extrapyramidal system – all motor parts of CNS except the pyramidal system.

Fasciculus – bundle of nerve fibres.

Ganglion – a swelling made up of nerve cells.

Gyrus – fold in the cerebral cortex.

Habenula – small swelling in the epithalamus.

Insula – hidden part of cortex in the lateral sulcus.

Ipsilateral – on the same side.

Lemniscus – bundle of nerve fibres in the CNS.

Neocortex – makes up most of cerebral cortex, 6 layers.

Pyramidal system – corticospinal and corticobulbar motor tracts that run in the pyramid shaped area in the medulla.

Sulcus – shallow grooves between gyri.

Neurochemistry

Neurotransmitters

Neurotransmitters (NT)

- Chemical substances present in neurone endings.
- Released at the synapse of a neurone in response to a stimulus.
- Attach to specific receptors on another neurone to produce a specific effect.
- Degraded by special mechanisms.

Transmitter synthesis

Method of synthesis depends on the neurotransmitter, see pharmacology of the neurotransmitters below:

Amino acids and amines

- Glutamate and glycine are amino acids found in all cells.
- Amines are only made in the neurones releasing them.
- Specific enzymes in the neurone convert precursor molecules into NT in the cytosol.

- The enzymes responsible for synthesis of amine NT are transported to the axon terminal producing local and rapid NT production.

Peptides

- Made in the cell body.
- Synthesised by the joining of amino acids by ribosomes in the rough endoplasmic reticulum.
- Cleaved in the Golgi apparatus to form the NT.
- Granules containing the NT bud off from the Golgi apparatus and are carried to the axon terminal by axoplasmic transport.

Transmitter storage and release

- Free NT is concentrated near nerve terminal.
- Taken up into synaptic vesicles for storage.
- Concentrated in the vesicle by transporter proteins in vesicle membrane.
- Action potential reaches axon terminal and triggers depolarisation of terminal membrane.
- Depolarisation causes voltage gated calcium channels to open and calcium to enter the cell.
- High concentration of calcium causes synaptic vesicles to fuse with presynaptic membrane and the proteins in vesicle membrane to change shape to form a pore releasing NT into the synaptic cleft.
- Membrane of synaptic vesicle becomes part of the presynaptic membrane and is later recovered by process of endocytosis.
- NT diffuses across synaptic cleft and activates postsynaptic receptors.
- Receptor activation may cause excitation or inhibition in the post-synaptic neurone.
- NT effects are actively ended by:
  - Clearance of transmitter.
  - Active uptake into presynaptic nerve terminal by selective carriers.
  - Active uptake into glial cells.
  - Degradation by local enzymes, e.g. ACh degraded by acetylcholine esterase
  - Modification of receptors.

A Synapse:

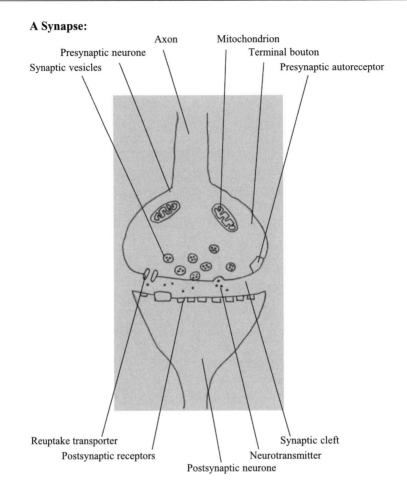

Basic pharmacology of the neurotransmitters

Dopamine (DA)

Precursor of noradrenaline. Brain DA originates from cell bodies in midbrain, neurones containing DA are clustered in the substantia nigra. DA pathways – main outputs are to the striatum and limbic system

- Nigrostriatal
- Mesocortical
- Mesolimbic

Synthesis and degradation:

- Produced from tyrosine a dietary amino acid.
- Tyrosine hydroxylase converts tyrosine to L-dopa – rate-limiting step.
- L-dopa is converted to dopamine by dopa decarboxylase.
- Stored in vesicles in the synaptic terminal and released when neurone depolarises.
- Taken back into nerve terminals or glial cells where it is metabolised by MAO-A.
- Metabolism also occurs outside neurones by MAO-B or catechol-O-methyl transferase (COMT) in the synaptic cleft to homovanillic acid (HVA) that can be used as an index of DA turnover.
- Some DA is used to make noradrenaline.

Functions:

- Voluntary movement – dysfunction can cause Parkinson's disease.
- Drive and reinforcement.
- Promotes nausea and vomiting.
- Role in schizophrenia and depression.

Noradrenaline (NA) or norepinephrine

Major catecholamine neurotransmitter in the CNS. Causes excitation in most cases but can be involved in inhibition. Noradrenergic neurones originate in the brainstem from the locus coeruleus and project to the cortex, cerebellum, hypothalamus and SC.
Synthesis and degradation:

- DA is transported into synaptic vesicles for conversion.
- NA is made from DA by the enzyme dopamine beta hydroxylase.
- This enzyme is present in the synaptic vesicles and is released with the NA.
- In vesicles the NA is joined to ATP which is released with the NT and may have NT properties itself.
- Some NA is actively pumped back into synaptic terminal where it is metabolised by MAO or recycled into vesicles.
- Metabolised by monoamine oxidase-A (MAO-A) to vanillomandelic acid (VMA) and 3-methoxy 4-hydroxylphenylglycol (MHPG).

Excitatory amino acids (EAA)

EAA include glutamate, aspartate and homocysteine. Main EAA is glutamate (glutamic acid):

• Made by the deamination of glutamine.
• Precursor to GABA.
• Widely distributed in the CNS.
• Involved in fast synaptic transmission, higher brain functions and plasticity.

Receptor structure and function

Receptors are membrane bound proteins that bind neurotransmitters and translate that molecular attachment to a physiological response. Amino acid sequences provide specificity for receptor binding. Divide receptors into 4 categories depending on mode of action and physiological response:

1. Receptors connecting to second messengers.
2. Receptors forming ion channels.
3. Receptors that attach to allosteric sites on other receptors.
4. Intraneuronal receptors.

Second messengers

The main second messengers are cyclic AMP, cyclic GMP, inositol triphosphate (IP3), diacyl glycerol (DAG) and arachidonic acid (AA). They mediate postsynaptic events and can be produced by the action of G proteins:

G proteins

Proteins in the membrane that can bind to the intracellular part of a receptor. NT can bind to receptors linked to excitatory or inhibitory G protein units. Excitatory units can activate enzymes including adenylate cyclase, guanylate cyclase, phospholipases C and A2 to produce the second messengers cAMP, cGMP, IP3/DAG and AA, respectively. These activate other cellular processes:

- Opening of ion channels.
- Activation of enzymes.
- Activation of calcium binding proteins.

Inhibitory subunits reduce the activity of the cyclase enzymes. G proteins can also control ion channels directly.

Ion channels

Ion channels are proteins found within the cell membrane and control cell excitability by allowing passage of electrical current through the membrane. Can be controlled (gated) by various factors including:

- Membrane potential.
- Neurotransmitters.
- Intracellular second messengers.

Abnormalities of ion channels can cause brain dysfunction. Selective channels exist for sodium, potassium, calcium and chloride:

Sodium channels

- Large protein that loops through cell membrane several times.
- Central channel/pore.
- Pore closed at resting membrane potential.
- Voltage gated; needs thousands of channels to generate an AP.

Potassium channels

- Protein spanning membrane similar to sodium and calcium channels.
- Triggered by several mechanisms:
  - Voltage change.
  - Calcium change.
  - Extracellular neurotransmitters.
  - Intracellular messengers.

Calcium channels

- 3 different types.
- Similar to sodium channels.
- Role in synaptic transmission and rhythmic firing of neurones.

Receptors for specific neurotransmitters

Dopaminergic receptors

Activated by dopamine. Originally classified 2 types – D1 and D2.
Other DA receptors have been identified, fall into 2 categories:

D1-like:
- Includes D1 and D5.
- Activates adenylate cyclase by G proteins.
- D1 is common in caudate, olfactory tubercle and nucleus accumbens.
- D5 is found outside striatum.

D2-like:
- Includes D2, D3 and D4.
- Inhibits adenylate cyclase by G proteins.
- D2 found in high levels in striatum.
- D2 blockade may cause extrapyramidal side effects of drugs.
- D3 found mainly in limbic areas.
- D3 presynaptic type of receptor may act as an autoreceptor.
- D4 found in limbic areas rather than striatum.

Noradrenergic receptors

Stimulated by noradrenaline. There are different classes of noradrenergic
receptors and subtypes of each class have been discovered:

Alpha-1:
- Postsynaptic receptors.
- Act via increasing phosphoinositol (PI) activity.
- Role in arousal.
- Blockade causes sedation and postural hypotension.

Alpha-2:
- Pre- and postsynaptic receptors.
- Act on G proteins and inhibits adenylate cyclase.
- Presynaptic alpha-2 receptors have a role in autoinhibition.
  - NA in synaptic cleft activates presynaptic receptors.
  - Presynaptic receptors increase potassium conductance and hyper-polarise cell.
  - Therefore inhibit further release of NA.
- Presynaptic alpha-receptor blockade facilitates NA release.
- Postsynaptic alpha-2 receptors affect release of growth hormone, arousal and blood pressure.

Beta:
- Coupled with G proteins and stimulate adenylate cyclase.
- β1 type are found mainly in the neurones and the heart.
- β2 type are dense in the cerebellum, tend to be found in glia and blood vessels.
- Presynaptic beta-receptor stimulation facilitates NA release.
- Role of β receptors is not clear.

Serotonergic receptors

At least seven classes exist with more subtypes identified depending on molecular properties and pharmacology. All except 5HT-3 are linked to G proteins.

5HT-1A receptors:
- Mainly autoreceptors, some postsynaptic receptors in hippocampus.
- Presynaptic receptor down-regulation causes antidepressant and anxiolytic actions.

5HT-1D receptors:
- Presynaptic autoreceptors at nerve terminal.
- Stimulation causes anti-migraine action.

5HT-2A receptors:
- Postsynaptic receptors, excitatory effect on cortical neurones.
- Receptor stimulation can cause anxiety, agitation, insomnia, akathisia and sexual dysfunction.

5HT-3 receptors:
- Stimulation can cause diarrhoea, nausea, headache.

GABA receptors

Several different classes:

GABA-A
- Form chloride selective channels.
- Found throughout the brain.
- Mediate fast synaptic inhibition in the brain.
- 5 subunits with central pore – different variations of subunits.
- Not open continuously in presence of GABA, flicker open and closed instead.
- Alpha subunit has a binding site for benzodiazepines.
- Benzodiazepines, barbiturates and anaesthetic steroids bind to GABA-A and enhance GABA activity.

- Benzodiazepines increase frequency of channel openings.
- Barbiturates prolong opening time of channel.
- Steroids increase opening time and frequency of opening.

GABA-B

- Slower acting.
- Less widely distributed in the brain.
- Presynaptically modulate NT release.
- Coupled to G proteins and modulate calcium or potassium channels.
- Often found on synaptic terminals where they inhibit NT release.

GABA-C

- Gate chloride channels.
- Mainly found in the retina.

Acetylcholine receptors

2 classes – nicotinic and muscarinic:

Nicotinic

- Ligand-gated ion channels.
- Fast acting, excitatory.
- Activation causes increased cellular permeability to sodium and potassium.
- Receptors vary in structure due to different subunits.
- Different combinations of subunits in different regions of brain.
- Present in the brain particularly the thalamus and cortex.

Muscarinic

- Slow acting.
- May be excitatory or inhibitory.
- Coupled to G proteins.
- Different subtypes – M1 to M5.

Excitatory amino acid receptors

Glutamate receptors. Divide into:

1) NMDA (N-methyl-D-aspartate) receptors.
   - Mainly postsynaptic.
   - Concentrated in the limbic system.
   - Act as ion channels to control calcium influx.
   - NMDA receptor blocked by magnesium at the resting potential of most neurones.

- To open the channels, membrane must depolarise to displace the magnesium.
- Needs glycine to bind simultaneously to activate channel and cause depolarisation.

2) AMPA receptors
- Gate sodium channels.
- Mainly postsynaptic.
- Responsible for most fast excitatory transmission.
- Wide distribution in cortex and ventral striatum.

3) Kainate receptors
- Gate sodium channels.
- Mainly presynaptic and regulate release of glutamate.
- Found in hippocampus mainly.

4) Metabotropic receptors – coupled to G proteins.

Pharmacology of neurotransmitters in relation to psychiatric disorders

Schizophrenia

DA, 5HT and glutamate are all implicated. Less evidence for ACh, NA and GABA.
DA theory supported by:

- Amphetamine – causes release of DA and produces similar symptoms.
- Antipsychotic drugs act via DA receptor blockade.
- Increased striatal D2 receptors found at post mortem and in functional imaging.
- Clozapine may have highest affinity for D4 receptors but it also acts on 5HT2, muscarinic and alpha-adrenergic receptors.

5HT theory:

- Hallucinogenic properties of LSD.
- Increased 5HT concentrations in basal ganglia at post mortem.
- Reduced 5HT2 receptors in prefrontal cortex.
- Increased 5HT2 and 5HT1A receptors in limbic cortex.
- Clozapine has high affinity for 5HT2A receptors.
- Possible abnormal CSF ratio of DA:5HT metabolites.

Roles:
- Controls the release of adrenocorticotrophic hormone (ACTH) from the anterior pituitary that stimulates the manufacture and release of adrenal cortical hormones (glucocorticoids).
- Reduces appetite and sexual drives.
- Excess amounts of CRH release linked with depression, panic attacks and alcohol withdrawal.
- CRH stimulates firing of noradrenergic neurones in locus coeruleus by affecting inhibition. CRH overactivity may therefore cause excess noradrenergic activity found in panic attacks and alcohol withdrawal.

Cholecystokinin (CCK)

Produced in the lining of the small intestine. Also found in the CNS – significance is unclear. High levels in cortex, hippocampus and amygdala. Coexists with substance P in the spinal cord.
Roles:
- May modulate DA pathway activity.
- May inhibit feeding.
- May have role in pain control.
- CCK in the gastrointestinal tract regulates release of bile after meals.

Substance P

Found in sensory neurones, spinal cord and areas of brain associated with pain. Conducts pain related nerve impulses from periphery to the CNS. Endorphins may act by suppressing its release.

Endogenous opioids

- There are 3 types: enkephalins, endorphins and dynorphins.
- Made from polypeptide precursors.
- 3 classes of opioid receptor:
  - Mu.
  - Delta.
  - Kappa.
- Each opioid type has different receptor affinities.
- Receptors are found in high concentrations in sensory, hypothalamic and limbic regions.

- Receptors facilitate inhibitory transmission in the brain – inhibit release of other NT and peptides.
- Coupled to G proteins.
- Roles:
  ○ Released in response to stress.
  ○ Control pain.
  ○ May reinforce behaviour by modulating DA release and therefore play a role in addiction.
- Opioid antagonists are used to treat opiate addiction.
- Addiction to weight loss in anorexia nervosa may be caused by excess endorphins produced by stress of starvation.
- Suggested role in depression and schizophrenia.

Enkephalins

- Concentrated in thalamus, hypothalamus and pathways that relay pain.
- Potent analgesics – inhibit pain by suppressing substance P.
- Receptor affinities: delta > mu > kappa.

Endorphins

- Concentrated in the pituitary gland.
- Inhibit pain by suppressing substance P.
- Receptor affinities: mu > delta > kappa.
- Linked to other functions:
  ○ Body temperature control.
  ○ Hormonal regulation – puberty, sex drive and reproduction.
  ○ Memory and learning.

Dynorphins

- Found in posterior pituitary, hypothalamus and small intestine.
- Stronger than beta-endorphin.
- Receptor affinities: kappa > mu > delta.
- Inhibit pain and involved in the registering of emotions.

Corticosteroids

Corticosteroids are steroid hormones that are secreted by the adrenal cortex. Made from cholesterol. Can be divided into 3 types:

Glucocorticoids

○ Cortisol and corticosterone.
○ Secretion controlled by ACTH from the anterior pituitary.
○ Plasma cortisol levels have a diurnal pattern – peak in morning before waking.
○ Help control body metabolism.
○ Maintain normal cardiovascular function.
○ Role in adapting to stress – cortisol release increases during stress.

Mineralocorticoids

○ Main one is aldosterone.
○ Maintains sodium and potassium balance and extracellular fluid volume.

Sex hormones

○ Mainly androgens.
○ Role in reproductive function.

Corticosteroid receptors

• Intracellular proteins with DNA binding area.
• Found in nucleus or cytosol of cells.
• Steroid molecule crosses cell membrane due to lipid solubility.
• Binds to receptor site and causes receptor to unfold.
• May move from cytosol to nucleus.
• Bind to specific region of nuclear DNA.
• Produce specific mRNA and synthesis of specific proteins.
• Newly made proteins produce cellular effects.
• Physiological response may take hours or days to develop.
• Many effects as different steroids activate different genes.

Neuropathology

Neuropathology of the dementias

Alzheimer's disease

Macroscopic

• Reduced brain weight.
• Cerebral atrophy – especially frontal and temporal lobes.

- Widened sulci.
- Enlarged third and lateral ventricles.

Microscopic

- Neuronal loss.
- Senile plaques:
  - Lots in cortex – hippocampus and amygdala.
  - Irregular shapes with silver staining core containing amyloid.
  - Outer ring of filamentous material including paired helical filaments.
  - Reactive microglia in disintegrating tissue of the plaques.
  - Astrocytes around edge.
- Neurofibrillary tangles:
  - Present in neuronal cell bodies especially pyramidal cells of hippocampus.
  - Flame shape.
  - Made of an abnormal phosphorylated type of Tau protein.
- Granulovacuolar degeneration.
  - Small vacuoles appear around a granule in the cytoplasm of the neurone.
- Hirano bodies:
  - Inclusion bodies.
  - Eosinophilic oval shape structures.
  - May result from abnormal configuration of microfilaments.
- Amyloid angiopathy – deposits of amyloid around small blood vessels.
- White matter changes – degeneration of axons, gliosis, and astrocyte hyperplasia.

Vascular dementia

Macroscopic

- Usually have normal sized brain.
- Arteriosclerosis – thickening and loss of elasticity of arterial walls.
- May have localised or generalised atrophy with dilated ventricles.
- Infarcts:
  - Size and location depend on the blood vessel affected.
  - May be singular or multiple.
- Softening in cortex.

Microscopic

- Hypertensive changes in blood vessels.
- Neuronal loss.
- Various stages of infarction:
  - Swelling of brain tissue.
  - Presence of inflammatory cells.
  - Presence of macrophages.
  - Astrocytosis.
  - Scar and cavity formation.
- White matter may have irregular patches of demyelination.

Lewy body dementia

Macroscopic

- Mild cortical atrophy.
- Ventricular enlargement.
- Pale substantia nigra and locus coeruleus.

Microscopic

- Neuronal loss.
- Lewy bodies.
  - Neuronal inclusions with a hyaline appearance.
  - Dark central dense core and a less intensely stained body.
  - Peripheral pale halo.
  - Present in cortex, substantia nigra and other brainstem nuclei.
- Some Alzheimer's disease type changes are also present.
- Senile plaques.
- Neurofibrillary tangles are relatively few.
- Minor vascular disease in about 30%.

Pick's disease

Macroscopic features

- Severe atrophy usually limited to frontal and temporal lobes.
- Thin gyri ('knifeblade atrophy').
- Loss of myelin in white matter of affected lobes.

- Dilated ventricles.
- Atrophy of subcortical grey structures particularly the caudate nucleus and putamen.

Microscopic features

- Neuronal loss – particularly in outer layers of affected cortex.
- Pick cells – swollen pyramidal cells in cortex.
- Pick bodies – silver staining inclusion bodies, contain smoothly contoured random filaments, lack the central core and halo of Lewy bodies.
- Hirano bodies and granulovacuolar changes may be seen.
- Senile plaques and neurofibrillary tangles not seen.

Creutzfeld–Jacob disease

Macroscopic

- May give no visible changes.
- May have minimal atrophy and some ventricular dilatation.

Microscopic

- Appearance varies.
- May have neuronal loss and proliferation of astrocytes.
- May accumulate an abnormal protease-resistant protein.
- Vacuoles in cytoplasm of neurones.
- Spongiosis – small cystic spaces in grey matter.
- Usually no senile plaques or neurofibrillary tangles.

AIDS dementia complex

Macroscopic

- Atrophy with dilated ventricles and widened sulci.
- Meninges may be thickened.

Microscopic

- Characteristic multi-nucleated cells.
- Collections of microglia.
- Astrocytosis and areas of demyelination.
- Changes occur mainly in white matter and subcortical grey structures.
- May be evidence of secondary infections, e.g. fungi, bacteria.

Acute organic conditions

Delirium

Many different causes of delirium but the clinical picture is similar. Considered to be a generalised dysfunction of higher brain functions. Particular areas associated with delirium are:

- Prefrontal cortex.
- Right cerebral hemisphere – particularly parietal and inferomedial temporoparietal regions.
- Subcortical nuclei – particularly thalamus and caudate on right side.

These areas are interconnected and link to the brainstem, basal ganglia and temporolimbic cortex. Due to the extensive connections of the thalamus, even a small lesion produces delirium.
Dysfunction of:

- Temporolimbic region may cause thought disorder, memory problems, delusions, hallucinations and illusions.
- Circuits linking basal ganglia and thalamus to prefrontal cortex may cause changes in personality, mood, motivation, and executive cognitive functions.
- Orbitofrontal region may cause disinhibition.

Neurochemical abnormalities:

- Changes in cholinergic and dopaminergic systems, which are also affected by serotonergic, opiatergic, GABAergic and glutamatergic systems.
- Neurotransmission may be altered by changes in general metabolism.
- Specific receptors and transmitters affected in different causes of delirium.

Anticholinergic hypothesis:

- Anticholinergic effects of medication produce delirium.
- Medical conditions produce delirium by reducing ACh by affecting glucose metabolism and the production of acetyl-coenzyme A (rate limiting step for ACh synthesis), e.g. hypoxia, hypoglycaemia, thiamine deficiency.

Dopaminergic hypothesis:

- Increased DA activity may occur due to reduced ACh activity.
- Dopaminergic drug toxicity causes delirium.
- Opiates cause release of DA and produce delirium.
- Hypoxia increases DA release.
- Hepatic encephalopathy produces excess DA.
- Mesolimbic and mesofrontal DA pathways may also be involved.

Other neurochemical changes:

- Increased GABA – hepatic encephalopathy.
- Reduced GABA – alcohol withdrawal, hypnotics.
- Increased serotonin – hepatic encephalopathy, sepsis, serotonergic syndrome.
- Serotonergic activity regulates DA activity in some parts of the brain.
- Suggested effects with reduced histamine, increased glutamate and increased cytokines.

Neuropathology of schizophrenia

Macroscopic findings

- Enlarged lateral and third ventricles.
- Decreased cortical volume affecting grey rather than white matter.
- Disproportionate loss from temporal lobe including hippocampus.
- Decreased thalamic volume.
- Enlarged basal ganglia secondary to antipsychotic medication.

Microscopic findings

- Absence of gliosis.
- Smaller cortical and hippocampal neurones.
- Fewer neurones in dorsal thalamus.
- Reduced synaptic and dendritic markers in hippocampus.
- Maldistribution of white matter neurones.
- Entorhinal cortex dysplasia.
- Cortical or hippocampal neurone loss.
- Disarray of hippocampal neurones.

Neuropathology of conditions associated with mental retardation

Autism

Macroscopic findings

- Little evidence of gross pathology at post mortem.
- CT/MRI – inconsistent findings include reversed cerebral asymmetries, enlargement of lateral and third ventricles, small cerebellar vermis, reduced radiodensity of the caudate, polymicrogyria.
- Association with widespread cerebral damage in cases of secondary autism, e.g. related to Tuberous Sclerosis, Phenylketonuria, etc.

Microscopic findings

- Alterations in cell packing in hippocampus and related limbic structures.
- Fewer purkinje cells in cerebellum.

Neurochemical findings

- Increased platelet 5HT in 30%.
- Increased DA in CSF.
- Reduced DA hydroxylase.
- Increased urinary and CSF HVA.
- Increased plasma NA.
- Increased opioid levels in CSF.
- Reduced plasma endorphin.
- Reduced nicotinic receptors in all brain areas.

Down's syndrome

- Small head.
- Simple brain structure.
- Low brain weight.
- Pre-senile dementia with cortical atrophy, amyloid plaques, neurofibrillary tangles and granulovacuolar degeneration.

Rett syndrome

- X-linked dominant progressive degenerative disorder.
- Normal development until about 18 months then progressive cortical atrophy and neuronal loss.

- Microcephaly, reduced cerebral volume.
- Greater loss of grey matter relative to white matter.
- Reduced blood flow in frontal cortex.
- Reduced DA activity in basal ganglia, substantia nigra and cortex.
- Reduced levels of metabolites of NA and DA in CSF.

Tuberous sclerosis

- Autosomal dominant inheritance or new mutations.
- Nodules (tubers) – hard, white, vary in size up to 3 cm, made of dense glial material.
- Appear over ventricular surfaces and sometimes on surface of cortex.
- May block circulation of CSF or become neoplastic.

Neuropathology of movement disorders

Parkinson's disease

Main pathological features:

- Degeneration and neuronal loss in the substantia nigra.
- May have diffuse cortical atrophy.
- Lewy bodies in areas with neuronal degeneration.
  - Substantia nigra.
  - Locus coeruleus.
  - Raphe nuclei.
  - Nucleus basalis of Meynert.
  - Thalamus.
  - Hypothalamus.
  - Autonomic nervous system.
  - Limbic cortex and cerebral neocortex.
- Loss of substantia nigra neurones causes loss of nigrostriatal dopaminergic innervation.
- This causes loss of the net inhibitory dopamine input to the striatum.
- Increases the inhibitory striatal input to the globus pallidus.
- Normal levels of GABA and glutamate are altered.
- Finally leads to loss of the normal thalamic excitatory stimulation of the cerebral cortex.
- Failure of appropriate thalamic stimulation of the supplementary motor cortex correlates with akinesia.

- Dopamine depletion more marked in the dorsal putamen than ventrally – correlates with the clinical presentation as the dorsal putamen represents the lower limbs and the ventral putamen the trunk and upper limbs.

Huntington's disease

Macroscopic findings

- Generalised cortical atrophy particularly in frontal lobes.
- Marked ventricular dilatation.
- Atrophy of the head of the caudate nucleus and the putamen.

Microscopic findings

- Marked loss of small nerve cells with relative preservation of larger motor cells in corpus striatum.
- Severe neuronal loss in outer cortex of the frontal lobes.
- Severe neuronal loss and astrocytic proliferation in the caudate and putamen.
- Neuronal fibre loss in white matter, corpus callosum may appear thin.
- Loss of striatal GABA neurones projecting from striatum to lateral part of globus pallidus or substantia nigra.

Tardive dyskinesias

- Pathogenesis yet to be clarified.
- No consistent finding at post mortem.
- Reports of microscopic changes in basal ganglia.
- Clinical picture may be caused by combination of:
  - Neuronal damage in basal ganglia.
  - Long term DA receptor blockade.
- DA receptor supersensitivity theory:
  - Postsynaptic DA receptors develop supersensitivity to antipsychotic drugs.
- Problems with theory:
  - Discrepancy between development of clinical picture and time of the increase in DA receptors following treatment.
  - All animals given antipsychotics develop receptor supersensitivity but only 20% of patients develop the persisting dyskinesia.
  - No TD seen in animals with increased receptor sensitivity.

○ Receptors return to normal after drug withdrawal but symptoms persist for years.

○ No difference in DA receptors post mortem for patients with and without TD.

• GABA theory:

○ Reduced GAD activity in parts of basal ganglia in animals on long-term antipsychotics – causes orofacial movements.

○ GABA agonists may improve some TD symptoms.

○ Patients with schizophrenia found to have lower levels of CSF GABA.

Relationship between localisation of cerebral damage and clinical signs

Different patterns of symptoms depend on the exact location of the lesion. Possible deficits include:

Frontal lobe

• Personality changes.
• Contralateral spastic paresis.
• Motor (expressive) dysphasia.
• Motor agraphia.
• Apraxia of face and tongue.
• Anosmia.
• Urinary incontinence.

Parietal lobe

• Conduction aphasia.
• Constructional and dressing apraxias.
• Dyslexia, dysgraphia and dyscalculia.
• Gerstmann syndrome – finger agnosia, dyscalculia, agraphia, right–left disorientation
• Anosagnosia, hemisomatagnosia, prosopagnosia, autopagnosia.
• Cortical sensory loss with astereognosis, agraphaesthesia, sensory inattention, impaired 2-point discrimination.
• Contralateral visual field defect.

Temporal lobe

• Sensory (receptive) dysphasia.
• Alexia, agraphia.

- Amnesic syndrome.
- Impaired learning and retention of verbal (dominant) or non-verbal (non-dominant).
- Personality disturbance.
- Contralateral homonymous upper quadrantic visual defect.

Occipital lobe

- Visual object agnosia or prosopagnosia.
- Visuo-spatial agnosia.
- Agnosia for written material.
- Homonymous visual defects.
- Cortical blindness.

Hypothalamus

Polydipsia, polyuria, hormonal changes, obesity, change in body temperature.

Thalamus

- Anterograde and retrograde amnesia.
- Impaired executive functions.
- Sensory deficits.
- Problems with attention and concentration.

Corpus callosum

- Apraxia to verbal commands.
- Agraphia and astereognosis.

Brain stem

- Cranial nerve palsies (pattern depends on level of lesion).
- Symptoms caused by damage to motor and sensory tracts.

Upper motor neurone lesion produces

- Spastic paralysis.
- Increased tone.
- Increased stretch reflexes.
- Babinski sign.

Lower motor neurone lesion produces

- Flaccid paralysis.
- Reduced tone.
- Reduced reflexes.
- Wasting, fibrillation and fasciculation.

Neuroimaging techniques

X-ray

- Shows bony abnormalities, calcification and some vascular abnormalities.
- Calcification of the pineal gland may show if there has been a shift of midline structures.
- Tumours may be calcified or cause erosion or overgrowth of bone.
- Aneurysms may also have calcified walls.

Computerised Axial Tomography

- Narrow beam of x-rays pass through body at many angles.
- Data absorption values calculated for different tissues.
- Presented as a series of transverse slices of cranial contents.
- Contrast can be used to enhance lesions.
- Image shows ventricles, sulci, thalami, head of caudate, internal capsule, optical radiations.
- Used to diagnose:
  - Space occupying lesions – tumours, abscesses, haematomas.
  - Cerebral atrophy.
  - Oedema.
  - Demyelinating disorders.

Positron Emission Tomography

- Uses short-lived radioisotopes that can be injected or inhaled.
- Isotopes emit positively charged particles in tissues and these particles release photons of energy when they join with electrons.
- A scanner can measure the photons and a computer creates a cross-sectional image of brain radioactivity.
- Used to assess density and affinity of neuroreceptors and measure blood flow and metabolic rates.

Single Photon Emission Computerised Tomography

- Similar to PET.
- Uses radiochemicals that emit single photons.
- These chemicals are taken up into the brain, and their concentration in different regions is measured by a rotating gamma camera that detects their energy.
- Cheaper than PET but image resolution less good.
- Used to measure cerebral blood flow or metabolism in different areas of the brain, e.g. reduced uptake in temporoparietal regions in Alzheimer's dementia.

Magnetic Resonance Imagery

- Patient placed in a strong magnetic field.
- Pulsed radio waves directed at brain tissue.
- Hydrogen nuclei in tissues align in same direction and resonate at same frequency as the stimulating radio frequency.
- Signals transformed by a receiver and computer into a visible scan.
- Signal varies depending on water content of tissue (e.g. bone has poor signal)
- Advantages
  - ○ Better resolution than CT particularly between white and grey matter.
  - ○ Imaging can be done in different planes.
  - ○ No ionising radiation used therefore safer.
  - ○ Functional MRI can be used to map brain areas involved in specific activities.
- Disadvantages
  - ○ Costly.
  - ○ Time consuming.
  - ○ Claustrophobic environment.
  - ○ Abnormalities of bone are not visualised.

Neurophysiology

Physiology of neurones

Characteristics of cell membranes

- Impermeable to large molecules, e.g. proteins.
- Permeable to water and lipophilic substances.

- Selective permeability to ions, e.g. potassium > sodium
- Act as if there were pores in the membrane.

Resting membrane potential

There is an electrical gradient between the outside and inside of the neuronal membrane. Occurs due to the distribution of ions (molecules with a net electrical charge). The distribution of ions causes a potential difference across the cell membrane.

- Potassium, phosphate and protein concentrations are higher inside the cell.
- Sodium and chloride concentrations are higher outside the cell.
- Resting potential of most neurones between −50 mV and −90 mV.

Ions move by diffusion down concentration gradients from high to low concentration. The sodium pump

- maintains these ionic gradients.
- is a protein present in the cell membrane.
- breaks down ATP and uses released energy to pump 3 sodium ions out of the cell in exchange for 2 potassium ions.
- creates a potential difference across the membrane of about −5 mV.

Action potential (AP)

The process of reversal of electrical charge across the neuronal membrane. Triggered by:

- opening of voltage gated sodium channels,
- action of neurotransmitters on channels, or
- electrical current.

Frequency of firing reflects the size of the depolarising current. Phases in the action potential:

- Rising phase − rapid depolarisation of membrane, membrane potential peaks at about +40 mV.
- Falling phase − rapid repolarisation of membrane.
- Hyperpolarisation − membrane potential more negative than resting potential.
- Gradual restoration back to resting potential.

- Absolute refractory period – a second AP cannot be triggered for about 1 msec after the first.
- Relative refractory period – requires a higher than usual current to depolarise the neurone to threshold level.

Action potential conduction:

- Depolarisation of membrane initiates an AP.
- Positive charge depolarises segment of membrane immediately next to it until it reaches threshold and generates its own AP.
- AP works down the axon until reaches axon terminal and initiates synaptic transmission.
- Conduction in one direction only because membrane behind the AP is refractory.
- AP can however begin from either end of neurone.

Ion fluxes during the action potential:

- Stimulus causes opening of sodium channels.
- Sodium enters neurone and causes depolarisation.
- If depolarisation reaches threshold an action potential will be generated.
- The positive charge of depolarisation causes sodium channels to close.
- Potassium channels remain open and potassium flows out of the cell due to the positive charge inside until resting membrane potential is reached.

Synapses:

- Synapses are specialised junctions that enable communication between neurones.
- Action potential opens voltage gated calcium channels in presynaptic terminal.
- Calcium enters the terminal and causes synaptic vesicles to fuse with presynaptic membrane.
- Vesicle releases neurotransmitters into synaptic cleft where they diffuse across the synaptic cleft to bind with postsynaptic receptors.
- Receptor activation causes either excitation or inhibition of the postsynaptic neurone.
- Action of neurotransmitter is ended by:
  - Diffusion away from the synaptic cleft.
  - Reuptake into the terminal or surrounding cells.
  - Breakdown by enzymes.

Synaptic integration:

- Neurones receive thousands of inputs.
- Inputs may be:
  - Excitatory – produce excitatory postsynaptic potentials (EPSP).
  - Inhibitory – produce inhibitory postsynaptic potentials (IPSP).
- Neurone has to integrate inputs, i.e. add up all EPSPs and IPSPs to see whether the final signal reaches threshold and will cause an AP.
- Part of axon nearest the cell body (axon hillock) has the lowest threshold and it is the integration of inputs here that usually determines if an AP will occur.
- Repeated stimulation of a single synapse can cause summation over time and reach threshold for neuronal firing.
- Stimulation of different synapses at the same time can also reach threshold level.

For synthesis, release and uptake of neurotransmitters refer to neurochemistry section.

Physiology and anatomical pathways of integrated behaviours

Perception

- The conscious registration of a sensory stimulus.
- For a sensation to occur there must be:
  - A stimulus.
  - A receptor to detect the stimulus.
  - Conduction of this information to the brain.
  - An area of the brain to transfer this information into a sensation.

Light touch and pressure

- Most sensory receptors in the somatic sensory system are mechanoreceptors.
- Present throughout the body.
- Mechanoreceptors have unmyelinated axon branches with ion channels that open in response to changes in tension of the membrane.
- Types of mechanoreceptor:
  - Pacinian corpuscle – deep in dermis, large receptive field, quick response, rapidly adapts.

○ Ruffini's endings – large receptive field, slowly adapting, sustained response.

○ Meissner's corpuscles – small receptive field (mm), quick response, rapidly adapts.

○ Merkl's discs – epidermis, small receptive field, slowly adapting, sustained response.

Pathway

- Stimulation causes deformation of membrane and opening of mechano-sensitive ion channels.
- Sufficiently large currents cause axon to fire an AP that is carried along primary afferent nerves.
- Enter spinal cord (SC) through dorsal roots – cell bodies lie in dorsal root ganglia.
- Decussate in SC.
- Information travels up spinal cord in the contralateral dorsal columns (anterior spinothalamic tract).
- Ascend in the medial lemniscus (white matter tract) through brainstem and synapse with neurones of the ventral posterior nucleus of the thalamus.
- Transformation of information takes place in the dorsal column and the thalamus.
- Thalamic neurones project to primary somatosensory cortex in post-central gyrus.
- Body areas can be mapped onto somatosensory cortex – sensory homunculus.
- Area of cortex devoted to each body part depends on density of sensory input for that part.

Vibration and position sense

- Vibration sensations are caused by the fast repetitive stimulation of touch receptors.
- Proprioceptive receptors are found in joints, skeletal muscles, tendons and the inner ear.
- Axons from both types of receptor enter dorsal columns of spinal cord.
- Ascend ipsilateral side in fasciculus gracilis and fasciculus cuneatus pathways.
- Decussate in medulla and form medial lemniscus.
- Pass to the thalamus and then on to the somatosensory area of cortex.

Temperature sensation

- Thermoreceptors detect either hot or cold sensation.
- Warm receptors are stimulated with temperatures >30°C until about 45°C when tissues burn. Receptors are coupled to C fibres.
- Cold receptors are stimulated by temperatures between 35 and −10°C. receptors are coupled to Aδ and C fibres.
- Pathway virtually identical to the pain pathway with information being carried in the lateral spinothalamic tract.

Pain

Pain is the perception of unpleasant sensations. Nociception is the sensory process that provides signals that trigger pain. Receptors (Nociceptors):

- Unmyelinated nerve endings that signal damage to body tissues.
- Present in most tissues but not the brain (except meninges).
- Activated by strong mechanical stimulation, extreme temperatures, oxygen deprivation, chemical exposure, etc.
- Individual nociceptors respond to different stimuli or some can be polymodal.

Stimulus causes opening of mechanically gated ion channels and depolarization of the cell, e.g.:

- Damaged cells can release substances that open ion channels.
- Proteases – break down extracellular peptides to form bradykinin that changes ion conductance of nociceptors.
- ATP – binds directly to ion channels of nociceptors.
- Potassium – increase in extracellular concentration of K^+ directly depolarises membrane.

Different fibres carry information of different types of pain:

- Aδ fibres – small myelinated fibres, carry well-localised fast sharp pain.
- C fibres – unmyelinated fibres, carry fibres for poorly localised, secondary, duller and longer-lasting pain.

Pathway:

- Pain afferents Aδ have cell bodies in dorsal root ganglia and enter dorsal horn of SC.
- Fibres may travel up or down SC for a short distance before synapsing in the substantia gelatinosa of the dorsal horn.

- Axons decussate in SC and travel in the lateral spinothalamic tract.
- Axons pass through brainstem and synapse in ventral posterior nucleus or intralaminar nuclei of the thalamus.
- Thalamus projects axons to primary somatosensory cortex.

Regulation of pain:

1. Activation of large mechanoreceptive afferents can reduce some types of pain, e.g. pain relief after trauma by rubbing skin.
2. Periaqueductal grey (PAG) neurones:
   - Inputs from brain areas involved in transmitting signals related to emotions.
   - Outputs to raphe nuclei that send projections down to dorsal horns of spinal cord.
   - Reduces activity of nociceptive receptors.
   - Stimulation of PAG causes analgesia.
3. Endogenous opioids:
   - Inhibit neurones by hyperpolarising postsynaptic membrane.
   - Suppress release of glutamate.
   - Endorphin containing neurones in SC and brainstem prevent passage of nociceptive signals through dorsal horn to higher levels of brain.

Memory

Memory is the ability to recall information. A change in the CNS represents a particular experience. This memory trace is known as an engram. Method of storage is unclear but possible theories on memory storage include changes in

- Electrical activity of neurones and their connections.
- Synapses between cells.
- Synthesis of NT and proteins.
- Neuronal gene expression.

Areas of brain involved vary depending on type of memory:

Declarative memory

- Memory for facts and events, available for conscious recollection.
- Involves medial temporal lobe, diencephalon.

- Medial temporal lobes:
  - Contain key structures including hippocampus, surrounding cortical areas and pathways connecting these parts with the rest of the brain.
  - Inputs come from association areas of cortex and contain highly processed information from all sensory modalities.
  - May consolidate memory into cortex but may do some intermediate processing.
- Diencephalon:
  - Anterior and dorsomedial nuclei of thalamus and mammillary bodies in hypothalamus implicated in processing of recognition memories.
  - Input from temporal lobe structures.
  - Lesions to both anterior and dorsomedial nuclei of the thalamus produce retrograde degeneration.
  - Lesions in medial temporal lobes and diencephalic lobes produce similar deficits and this suggests that these interconnected areas are part of a system serving a common function of memory consolidation.
  - Hippocampal lesions produce working memory deficits.

Non-declarative memory

- Procedural memory for skills, habits and behaviours involves the striatum.
- Classical conditioning for emotional responses involves the amygdala, and for skeletal muscle it involves the cerebellum.

Motor function

Motor cortex receives inputs from:

- Premotor cortex – plans movement, particularly complex movements of distal muscles.
- Posterior parietal cortex – uses somatosensory, proprioceptive and visual inputs to generate a picture of body's position and relation in space.
- Basal ganglia – select and initiate movements.
- Cerebellum – movement sequences, co-ordination and accuracy.

Pathway:

Axons from primary motor cortex descend spinal cord in 2 groups of pathways:

Lateral pathways – corticospinal, rubrospinal:

- Control voluntary movements and are under direct cortical control.
- Corticospinal tract
  o Originate in motor cortex and some fibres from somatosensory cortex.
  o Fibres pass through internal capsule, midbrain and pons.
  o Form tract at base of medulla.
  o Tract forms bulge in surface of medulla = pyramidal tract.
  o Most fibres in the tract decussate at junction of medulla and spinal cord.
  o These axons collect in lateral column of spinal cord and form lateral corticospinal tract.
  o Axons end in dorsolateral region of ventral horns where motor neurones and interneurones for distal muscles lie.
  o The remaining axons travel in the anterior corticospinal tract on the ipsilateral side and decussate in the anterior grey horn of SC.
- Rubrospinal tract
  o Originates in red nucleus of midbrain that receives input from frontal cortex.
  o Almost immediately decussate in pons and join fibres in corticospinal tract.

Ventromedial pathways – reticulospinal, vestibulospinal, tectospinal:

- Use sensory information about balance, body position and visual environment to maintain balance and body posture.
- Control of postural muscles and locomotion, under brainstem control.
- Vestibulospinal tract
  o Originate in vestibular nuclei of medulla that relay sensory information from the ear.
  o Part of tract projects bilaterally down spinal cord to cervical spinal neurones that control muscles to guide head movement.
  o Other part projects ipsilaterally to lumbar spinal cord to facilitate extensor motor neurones of the legs.
- Tectospinal tract
  o Originates in superior colliculus of midbrain that receives visual, somatosensory and auditory inputs.
  o Controls posture of head and neck.

- Reticulospinal tract
  - Arises from reticular formation in pons and medulla.
  - Controlled by cortical signals.
  - Pontine reticulospinal tract facilitates extensors of lower limbs, maintains standing posture.
  - Medullary reticulospinal tract has opposite effect, frees these muscles from reflex control.

Role of the basal ganglia

See pages 97–99 for review of anatomy of the basal ganglia.

- Basal ganglia select and initiate willed movements.
- They receive inputs from frontal and parietal cortex.
- Globus pallidus cells are spontaneously active and have inhibitory effect on ventral lateral nucleus of the thalamus (VLN).
- Cortex provides excitatory input to the putamen.
- Putamen cells have inhibitory action on neurones in globus pallidus.
- VLN cells are released from inhibition and stimulate cortical activity in motor areas.

$$\text{Resting state:} \quad \text{GP} \xrightarrow{\text{Inhibits}} \text{VLN} \xrightarrow{\text{Unable to stimulate}} \text{Motor cortex}$$

$$\text{Movement:} \quad \text{Cortex} \xrightarrow{\text{Stim}} \text{Putamen} \xrightarrow{\text{Inhibits}} \text{GP} \xrightarrow{\text{Stops inhib}}$$

$$\text{VLN} \xrightarrow{\text{Stimulates}} \text{Motor cortex}$$

Role of the cerebellum

- Involved in sequencing of movement, co-ordination and accuracy.
- Essential for execution of planned, voluntary, multi-jointed movements.
- Cerebellum appears to instruct motor cortex with respect to movement direction, timing and force.
- Axons from sensorimotor cortex, somatosensory areas and posterior parietal areas project to nuclei in the pons.
- Pontine nuclei send information to the cerebellum.
- Lateral cerebellum sends projections to cortex via VLN of thalamus.

Drives

Motivation

- Motivation is the driving force on behaviour.
- Motivated behaviours generated by somatic motor system are made to occur by activities of the lateral hypothalamus, e.g. temperature regulation, thirst, and hunger.
- Mesocorticolimbic dopaminergic system may play important role in motivating behaviours.
- Areas found to be involved in reinforcement behaviours in experiments include:
  - Hypothalamus.
  - Septal nuclei.
  - Cingulated cortex.
  - Hippocampus.
  - Median forebrain bundle.

Sexual behaviour

- The amygdala is important in the regulation of sexual behaviour.
- Amygdala lesions cause hypersexuality.
- Septal lesions cause hyposexuality.
- Anterior hypothalamic lesions prevent hormonal activation of sexual activity.

Feeding

- Long-term regulation involves hormonal and hypothalamic regulation of body fat and feeding.
- Leptin is a hormone released by adipocytes.
- Changes in leptin levels are detected by the arcuate nucleus of the hypothalamus which projects axons to parts of the nervous system to co-ordinate a response – lateral hypothalamus, anterior pituitary and ANS.
- ↓ leptin causes:
  - Inhibition of TSH and ACTH.
  - Activation of parasympathetic system and stimulation of feeding behaviour.
- Bilateral lesions of lateral hypothalamus cause anorexia.

Inhibition of feeding:

- Leptin molecules are released into the blood by fat cells.
- Activates receptors on neurones of the arcuate nucleus of hypothalamus.
- Causes increased TSH secretion and increased ACTH.
- Results in increased metabolic rate and less feeding behaviour.

Short-term regulation of feeding:

- During absorption period, satiety signals → inhibit feeding.
- Gastric distention (detected by vagal neurones acting on medulla) → inhibit feeding.
- Food → release CCK → acts on vagal neurones.
- Insulin release acts directly on arcuate and ventromedial nuclei of hypothalamus.

Drinking

2 signals stimulate drinking:

1. Hypovolaemia (reduction in blood volume)
   - Reduced renal blood flow → release of angiotensin II → stimulates release of vasopressin from hypothalamus.
   - ↓ BP detected by receptors in blood vessels and heart → stimulus of vagus nerve → send signals to hypothalamus.
   - ↓ blood volume → stimulates sympathetic ANS → constriction of arterioles and motivation to seek water (lateral hypothalamus).
2. Hypertonicity (increase in concentration of solutes)
   - Sensed by lamina terminalis of the telencephalon.
   - Change in firing frequency of neurones → release of vasopressin and stimulate osmometric thirst.

Temperature regulation

Increased body temperature:
   - Detected by warm sensitive neurones of anterior hypothalamus.
   - Causes decreased TSH release, increased parasympathetic activity, panting and seeking cold.
Reduced body temperature:
   - Detected by cold sensitive neurones of anterior hypothalamus.
   - Causes increased TSH release with increased T4 and increased metabolic rate.

- Increased sympathetic activity with constricted blood vessels and piloerection.
- Shivering and seeking warmth.

Emotions

Aggression:
Aggression can be provoked by stimulation of:

- Amygdala
  - Acts as a gate to the limbic system, threatening stimuli can be evaluated.
  - Outputs to hypothalamus and limbic forebrain structures.
- Hypothalamus.
- Area around fornix.
- Ventral posterior lateral nucleus of thalamus.

Catecholamines may moderate threshold of incoming stimuli.
Aggressive behaviour facilitated by:

- Reduced 5HT and GABA.
- Increased ACh and catecholamines.

Fear:

- Feared stimulus causes activation of the amygdala.
- Amygdala neurones send axons to the central nucleus.
- Central nucleus sends projections to:
  - Hypothalamus which alters activity of ANS.
  - Periaqueductal grey matter in the brain stem that can evoke behavioural reactions via the somatic motor system.
  - Cerebral cortex which produces the emotional experience.

Anxiety:

- Septohippocampal circuit may modulate anxiety responses.
- Stimulation of septal area causes anxiety.
- Lesions of septal area and hippocampus cause behaviour similar to effects of anxiolytics.
- Septohippocampal circuit may act with Papez's circuit to make predictions about anticipated events and match them to real events.
- Differences between these can interrupt behaviour and increase arousal and attention.

Stress:

- Stress – psychological, physiological or emotional stimulation.
- Parvocellular neurosecretory cells in the hypothalamus determine whether a stimulus is stressful.
- Cause release of CRH → anterior pituitary produces ACTH → cortisol release from adrenal cortex.

Neurodevelopmental models of psychiatric disorders

Schizophrenia

Theory suggests:

- 'Brain lesions' originate in early life and predispose to the development of schizophrenia in later life.
- Genetic and environmental factors may produce these lesions.
- Evidence of abnormalities in childhood – lower IQ, impaired motor, cognitive and social skills.
- Lesions may only show later in life because normal brain maturation may need to occur before the problems are revealed.
- Supported by neuropathological findings (p. 135); lack of glial proliferation implies neurodevelopmental, not neurodegenerative, illness.
- Reduced reelin (protein helping neuronal migration and brain development) in some patients with schizophrenia.
- Recently identified gene Disrupted in Schizophrenia-1 (DISC-1), role in brain development, abnormalities may cause susceptibility to schizophrenia.

Autism

Evidence for a neurodevelopmental disorder:

- Perinatal origins.
- Link to viral and immune factors.
- Association with brain dysfunction – hippocampus, amygdala and cerebellum.
- Dopamine and serotonin abnormalities.
- Spectrum of neurobehavioural abnormalities.
- Mechanisms by which environmental triggers interact with developing immune and neural systems are poorly understood.

Evidence to support theory of viral infection:

- Retrospective epidemiological studies of in utero or perinatal viral exposures.
- Seasonal geographic factors.
- Studies of immune abnormalities in blood of autistic children.
- Expression may need presence of specific genes, an environmental trigger and the exposure to occur at a particular time during brain development.

Cerebral plasticity

- Cerebral plasticity is the re-organisation of connections between neurones.
- Functional recovery often follows damage.
- The function of the damaged area is taken over by other areas that have not been damaged.
- Structural changes occur with surviving pre-terminal axons growing new branches.
- These can form synapses at the sites denervated by the lesion.
- May be part of a normal process used in the learning of repetitive tasks.

Development and localisation of cerebral functions

Development of the nervous system begins early in the third week of development:

- Ectoderm thickens to form the neural plate.
- Neural plate folds to form longitudinal neural groove.
- The raised edges of the neural groove enlarge and meet to form the neural tube.

The wall of the neural tube has 3 layers:

- Outer marginal layer which forms white matter of the NS.
- Middle mantle layer which forms grey matter of the NS.
- Inner ependymal layer which forms lining of the ventricles.

The tissue between the neural tube and ectoderm differentiates to form:

- Spinal nerves, cranial nerves and their ganglia.
- Adrenal medulla and ganglia of ANS.

At 3–4 weeks the anterior part of the neural tube develops into 3 primary vesicles. By week 5 the vesicular region bends to form secondary vesicles.

Primary vesicle	Secondary vesicle	Final structure
Forebrain (prosencephalon)	Anterior telencephalon	Cerebral hemispheres Basal ganglia
	Posterior diencephalon	Thalamus Hypothalamus Pineal gland
Midbrain (mesencephalon)	Unchanged	Midbrain
Hindbrain (rhombencephalon)	Anterior metencephalon	Pons Cerebellum
	Posterior myelencephalon	Medulla

Area of neural tube posterior to the myelencephalon forms the spinal cord.

Effects of injury at different stages

Intrauterine period:

- Failure of the neural tube to close produces neural tube defects including anencephaly and spina bifida.
- Maximal neuronal proliferation occurs in the mid-trimester of pregnancy and is vulnerable to infection, radiation, drugs and alcohol.

Glial multiplication and myelination occurs up to 2 years of age and is potentially vulnerable to damage:

- Malnutrition can cause reduced neural connections by interfering with the formation of dendritic trees and synapse formation.
- Inborn errors of metabolism, toxins and environmental influences cause their most harmful effects during this period of fastest developmental change.
- Brain damage or malformation in early life produces cerebral palsy if it affects areas involved in motor function.

Brain damage after the developmental period produces the lesions listed on page 139 of the neuropathology section.

Neuroendocrine system

The neuroendocrine system

- co-ordinates the endocrine system, behaviour and development.
- involves the pituitary gland and the hypothalamus.

Pituitary gland

- A small gland that sits below hypothalamus and is connected to it by a stalk.
- Consists of 2 lobes – anterior and posterior.
- Controlled by the hypothalamus and the secretions of its own target glands.

Anterior pituitary

The anterior pituitary secretes a number of hormones that are made by different cell types in the AP:

Hormone	Function
Follicle stimulating hormone FSH	Ovulation/spermatogenesis
Luteinising hormone LH	Ovarian or sperm maturation
Thyroid stimulating hormone TSH	Thyroxine secretion by thyroid
Adrenocorticotrophic hormone ACTH	Stimulates adrenal cortex to secrete cortisol
Growth hormone GH	Growth and metabolism
Prolactin PRL	Stimulates/sustains lactation

- These hormones are secreted in response to stimulation by specific neurohormones that are made in the hypothalamus, released and diffuse into a capillary plexus.
- They are transported down large portal vessels in the pituitary stalk to a second set of capillaries in the anterior pituitary = hypophyseal portal system.

- The neurohormones act as releasing and inhibitory factors.
- Some of the AP hormones may be under dual control:

Hypothalamic releasing/ inhibitory factors	Function
Thyrotrophin releasing hormone TRH	Stimulates release of pituitary TSH Stimulates prolactin release
Gonadotrophin releasing hormone GnRH	Stimulates LH release Stimulates FSH release to lesser extent
Growth hormone releasing hormone GHRH	Stimulates release of GH
Growth hormone inhibitory hormone GHIH (somatostatin)	Inhibits release of GH
Corticotrophin releasing factor CRF	Stimulates release of pro-opiocortin peptides (ACTH)
Dopamine DA	Inhibits release of prolactin

Hypothalamic secretion of releasing and inhibitory factors may be influenced by emotional and environmental factors. Long-term regulation occurs through negative feedback loops:

- By the blood level of the anterior pituitary hormone.
- By the target gland.

Posterior pituitary

Posterior pituitary cells release 2 neurohormones – oxytocin and antidiuretic hormone. Made in supraoptic and paraventricular nuclei of the hypothalamus. Transported down axons to terminals in the posterior pituitary where they are stored until release.

1) Oxytocin
   - Released in final stages of childbirth.
   - Facilitates delivery by causing uterus to contract.
   - Stimulates ejection of milk from mammary glands.
2) Antidiuretic hormone ADH (vasopressin)
   - Release stimulated by changes in blood volume and salt concentration detected by receptors in the cardiovascular system and hypothalamus.
   - ADH acts on kidney to retain water and reduce urine production.

- Kidney itself detects low blood volume and pressure.
- Secretes renin which stimulates synthesis of angiotensin II by liver.
- Angiotensin II excites subfornical organ in telencephalon that stimulates hypothalamus to increase ADH production and thirst.

Main hormonal changes in psychiatric disorders

Depression

- Increased hypothalamic CRF.
- Increased secretion of cortisol in about 50% of depressed patients.
- Increased urinary free cortisol.
- Impaired suppression of cortisol by dexamethasone in about 50% of depressed in-patients.
- Reduced response of ACTH to CRF.
- Blunted TSH response to TRH in 20–70% patients.
- Increased TRH secretion and increased CSF TRH concentration.
- Abnormal GH regulation.
- Reduced concentration of somatostatin in CSF.
- Blunted GH response to insulin tolerance test.
- Blunted PRL responses.

Schizophrenia

- Inconsistent findings – less studied than depression.
- May have dexamethasone non-suppression.
- May have abnormal ACTH and cortisol responses to CRH.
- Reduced somatostatin in CSF.
- Reduced nocturnal GH secretion may occur.

Anorexia nervosa

- Hypercortisolism.
- Increased plasma GH.
- Menstrual disturbance – impaired gonadotrophin secretion, low oestradiol.
- Low total T4, normal free T4, low T3.
- Impaired osmotic regulation of vasopressin.

Alzheimer's disease

- May have reduced responsiveness of neuroendocrine systems influenced by cholinergic mechanisms.

- May have increased serum cortisol levels.
- May show dexamethasone non-suppression.
- May have reduced somatostatin in CSF and brain.

Neuroendocrine rhythms

- Humans have a fairly constant 24 hour rhythm of sleeping and waking = circadian rhythm.
- Physiological and biochemical processes vary with daily rhythms:
  - Growth hormone levels are highest during sleep.
  - Temperature drops slightly during sleep.
  - Cortisol levels are highest just prior to waking.
- Disrupted by shift work and jet lag.
- Suprachiasmatic nuclei (SCN) in the hypothalamus act as a biological clock.
- Axons from retinal cells synapse on SCN neurones.
- SCN sends signals to parts of the diencephalon.
- Lesions to these pathways cause disruption of the circadian rhythm.

Physiology of arousal and sleep

The reticular formation is a network of neurones extending throughout the brainstem. Receives inputs from sensory, visual, auditory and vestibular pathways. Sends projections to:

- Motor neurones of SC via reticulospinal tracts.
- Thalamus via the hypothalamus where inputs arrive from the limbic system.

The reticular formation and its connections with the thalamus are known as the ascending reticular activating system (ARAS). Arousal and consciousness are related to tonic control of ARAS. Other projections contributing to ARAS are from:

1) Locus coeruleus:
   - Noradrenergic nucleus in the pons.
   - Axons innervate nearly every part of the brain.
   - Involved in regulation of attention, arousal and sleep wake cycles.
   - NA makes neurones more responsive to stimuli.
   - LC may increase brain responsiveness, increase speed of information processing, increase efficiency.

2) Raphe nuclei:
- 9 nuclei lie either side of the midline of the brainstem.
- Contain serotonergic neurones that project to different areas of the brain.
- Fire rapidly when awake, aroused and active.

During sleep or relaxed waking:

- Reticulospinal tracts reduce skeletal muscle tone and sensitivity of reflexes.
- Rhythmic discharge of neurones in thalamus produces characteristic alpha and delta rhythms on EEG.

Sleep ends when sensory inputs and limbic system send signals to the reticular formation, e.g. if hungry/thirsty.

- Reticulospinal tracts stop inhibition of skeletal muscles.
- Reticular formation signals thalamus to block rhythmic brain activity.
- Cortex is free to respond to external environment and cognitive processing.

Stimulation of ARAS causes behavioural arousal and EEG desynchronisation. Lesions of ARAS cause permanent sleep. However, lesions within median raphe nuclei cause permanent insomnia.

Sleep

Sleep cycles every 90 minutes between different stages throughout night. 75% of sleep is non-REM, 25% REM. Progressive decrease in non-REM and increase in REM sleep as night progresses. REM cycles last 30–50 minutes with 30 minutes between periods. Half of REM sleep occurs in the last third of the night.

Stages of sleep:

	Awake	Alpha and beta rhythms
	REM	Beta rhythms
Stage 1	Drowsy	Theta rhythms
Stage 2	Light sleep	8–14 Hz sleep spindles and k complexes
Stage 3	Deep sleep	Delta rhythms
Stage 4	Deep sleep	Delta rhythms, 2 Hz or less

EEG

- Pictures electrical activity of cerebral cortex.
- Electrodes are taped over scalp.
- Small voltage fluctuations can be measured between selected pairs of electrodes.
- Thousands of neurones need to be activated simultaneously to generate a detectable signal.
- Amplitude of signal depends on synchronicity of underlying neurones.
- Signal varies depending on:
    o conscious level.
    o degree of mental activity.
    o pathology.
- Abnormal activity may be provoked by hyperventilation, sleep deprivation or photic stimulation.

Different types of brain waves

Alpha	8–13 Hz	Awake, resting with eyes shut, disappear in sleep
Beta	14–30 Hz	Mental activity, processing sensory input
Theta	4–7 Hz	Normal in children, stressed adults, some brain disorders
Delta	1–4 Hz	Normal in awake infant, adults in deep sleep, brain damage

Evoked responses

Evoked potentials are EEG waves elicited by repetitive stimulation of a single sensory pathway:

- Visual – 5% of patients with epilepsy respond to photic stimulation.
- Auditory.
- Somatosensory.

Changes in the waveforms of evoked potentials are used to diagnose some diseases, e.g. multiple sclerosis. P300 potential occurs 300 msec after the stimulus and can be abnormal in some psychiatric illnesses:

- Significantly delayed in patients with dementia.
- Most studies of schizophrenia have found reduced amplitudes of response with or without abnormal latencies.

Investigational uses

An abnormal EEG can suggest abnormal brain function but cannot make a diagnosis alone. A normal EEG does not exclude pathology.

Pathology	EEG pattern
Tonic clonic seizures	Generalised large 8–12 Hz spikes in groups during clonus
Absence seizures	Generalised 3 Hz spike and wave pattern
Partial seizures	Localised spikes or sharp waves
Schizophrenia	Non-specific patterns reported
Depression	'Reversal' of normal sleep EEG, reduced REM onset
Alzheimer's disease	Reduced alpha activity; diffuse theta or delta rhythms may appear
Huntington's disease	'Flattened' trace
CJD	Bilateral 3 Hz waves; or may have triphasic sharp wave complexes
Multi-infarct dementia	Some reported focal activity
Pick's disease	Some reduced frontal activity
Delirium	Slow alpha and generalised increase in delta waves
Space occupying lesion	Focal delta waves
Psychopathy	No characteristic pattern, 'immature' posterior temporal slow waves

Effects of drugs on EEG

Drug	Action
Neuroleptics	Increased theta and delta activity, reduced seizure threshold
Tricyclic antidepressants	Increased theta and delta activity, reduced seizure threshold
Hypnotics/sedatives	Increased beta activity particularly frontal area
Alcohol	Increased theta waves becoming delta waves, paroxysms on sudden withdrawal

6 | Social sciences

Sociology

Weber (1864–1920)

- Sociology as a comprehensive science of social action.
- Humans attach their actions and interactions within specific social contexts.
- *Social actions* (4 types) – zweckrational (rationally chosen), wertrational (value-oriented rationality), affective action (based on emotional state) and traditional action (i.e. guided by custom or habit).
- *Ideal type* – typical or 'logically consistent' features of social institutions or behaviour. An analytical construct that served for measuring the extent to which concrete social institutions are similar.
- *Bureaucracy* – a distinctive mark of modern social structure is the bureaucratic co-ordination of human actions. It is designed according to rational principles in order to efficiently achieve their goals. Characteristics of ideal-type bureaucracy:
  - Hierarchy of authority – information flowing up chain of command.
  - Impersonality.
  - Written rules of conduct.
  - Promotion based on achievement.
  - Division of labour.
  - Efficiency.

  Advantages: efficiency and achievement of goals.

  Disadvantages: impersonal and dehumanising. Unregulated social power.
- *Authority* – 3 main types:
  - Traditional authority – e.g. invested in a particular office by a higher power. Dominates in pre-modern societies.
  - Rational–legal authority – based on impersonal rules established legally. Dominates in modern societies.

  o Charismatic – appeal to leaders who command allegiance due to their unusual personalities.
- *Causality*
  o Multi-causality of social phenomenon.
  o Impossibility of making comprehensive predictions.
  o Prediction is only possible within a system of theory on a selection of social forces.
  o Contrary to Marx, Weber believed that both ideas and material factors are important determinants of social structure.
- *Protestant ethic*
  o Modern society is characterised by rational actions in a system with rational–legal authority.
  o Weber focused on the shift from traditional to rational action.
  o The protestant ethic provides religious sanctions for a spirit of rigorous discipline and to apply them rationally to acquire wealth.
  o It is a powerful force for the development of capitalism.
- *Oligarchy*
  o Rule by a few officials at the top of the organisation.
  o Results from bureaucracy.
  o Self-appointed leaders may control quality of our lives.
- *Societal oligarchy*
  o Oligarchy within whole societies.
  o Bureaucrats are needed to control and co-ordinate complex societies.
  o However, this also undermines freedom and democracy.
  o Government's responsibility to the electorate does not really exist, as people do not even know who the bureaucrats are or what they are doing.
- *Rationalisation and the irrationality factor*
  o Rationalisation – practical application of knowledge to achieve desired end. Leads to efficiency, control, co-ordination and increased productivity.
  o Basic principle behind division of labour and bureaucracy
  o However, even though rational thinking in bureaucracy leads to increased efficiency, it is not necessarily morally rational. What is good for the bureaucracy is not necessarily good for the society as a whole.
  o Hence, bureaucracies may paradoxically act in very irrational ways.

Marx

- *Marxism* – Theory put forwarded by Marx and Engels. Theory of 'dialectical materialism' based on *communist* practice.
- *Materialism* – Humans depend on the material world. It starts with the real process of production as the basis of all history. All different theoretical products and forms of consciousness arise from it.
- *Capital* – Capitalistic exploitation results from the extraction of the difference between the cost of a product and the cost of production. It is created from labour power.
- *Class formation* – In the process of production, humans work with one another. When humans organised themselves according to the division of labour, classes in society formed based on the different roles and positions the people found themselves in. Examples of classes are the proletariat (i.e. labourers) and the bourgeois.
- *Class struggle* – With the advancement of productive forces, workers in one class (e.g. manual labourers) can become redundant and are forced out (e.g. in Industrial Revolution). Bourgeois society built up enormous means of production and exchange as capital. Increasing improvement of machinery makes livelihood of workmen more precarious. Collision between individual workmen and bourgeois develop into a class struggle.
- *The Socialist revolution* – The proletariat must wrest all capital from the bourgeois and centralise all instruments of production in the hands of the state. For example, there may be
  - Abolishing land ownership.
  - Heavy and progressive income tax.
  - Abolishing rights of inheritance.
  - Centralisation of banks, communications, transport, and factories.
  - Equal obligation of all to work.
- *Communists* – People who actively support the interests of the working class. The immediate aim is to form the proletariat into a class, overthrow the bourgeois supremacy and the proletariat conquest of political power.

Durkheim (1858–1917)

4 major works: The Division of Labour in Society (1893), The Rules of Sociological Method (1895), Suicide (1897) and The Elementary Forms of the Religious Life (1912).

Division of labour in society

Following Adam Smith's economic principles on division of labour and utilitarian principle of maximisation of happiness, Durkheim addresses 3 questions about it

- *What is its function?*
  - Division of labour has no role other than to render civilisation. However, since crimes and suicide increase with civilisation, civilisation is at best morally indifferent.
  - The real function of division in labour is not economical, but to create a feeling of solidarity in 2 or more persons.
  - Modern individuals receive from society all that is necessary for life, and therefore creates strong sentiment of personal dependence.
  - Society also learns to regard its members not as homogeneous units, but as irreplaceable parts. Social evolution occurs by the perfection of such moral function.
- *What are the causes?*
  - Durkheim did not believe that division in labour could have resulted from a desire for happiness, and was doubtful that the advance of civilisation caused happiness anyway.
  - Further such 'happiness' theory could not account for the non-existence of division of labour in some societies.
  - Disappearance of the segmental structure may cause division of labour, or vice versa.
- *Abnormal forms of the division of labour* – 3 abnormal forms
  - Individuals increasingly become more isolated by their more specialised task (anomie division of labour).
  - Forced division of labour.
  - Lack of continuity – one organ can do more only if other organs do more.
- *Principles of ethics* – those that internalise the conscience collective of the groups we belong to. The moral quality is derived from the essential function in preventing social disintegration.

The rules of sociological method

Durkheim claimed that these methods are 'free of political and philosophical doctrine'.

1) *Social Fact*
  o Durkheim distinguished between 'states of the collective mind' from those manifested through individual minds.
  o He recommended the use of statistics to 'cancel out' influence of individual cases.
  o May be recognised by the presence of external sanctioning.
  o Include both ways of functioning (e.g. acting, thinking) and being (e.g. the number, geographical location, relation to other members of society).
2) *Rules for observations of social fact*
  o Treat social facts as things
  o Systematically discard all preconceptions
  o Subject matter must only include a pre-defined group of phenomena
  o Consider only from the viewpoint where social facts present themselves
3) *Rules for distinguishing the normal from the pathological*
  o A social fact is normal for a given social type when it occurs in the average society of that species.
4) *Rules for the explanation of social facts*
  o To explain a social phenomenon, the efficient cause which produces it and the functions it fulfils must be investigated separately.
  o The determining cause of a social fact must be sought amongst the antecedent social facts and not among the states of the individual consciousness.
  o The function of a social fact must be sought in relation to the social end it bears upon.
5) *Rules for the Demonstration of Sociological Proof*
  o Experimentation – when 2 phenomena are produced artificially.
  o Comparative method (compare phenomena produced naturally) – but not all forms of this method can be applied to studying social facts.

Suicide

1) *Definition*
  o The distinctive feature is not that it is performed intentionally, but advisedly (i.e. knows the consequences of the result).
2) *Extra-social Causes*
  o Possible causes: individual psychological constitution and external physical environment.

○ Annual rate of suicide is relatively stable for a given society.
○ Durkheim noted that many suicides are not connected with insanity.
○ He noted that suicide increases in those months, days of the week and hours of the day when social life is most active. Hence, suicide reflects the consequence of the intensity of social life.

3) *Egoistic suicide*
○ Lower rates of suicide in religious groups, more so in Catholics than Protestants. Durkheim attributed this to the greater degree of free inquiry permitted in Protestants which is in turn due to its fewer commonly accepted beliefs and practices.
○ Amongst other societies (e.g. family, political), only marriage has a preventive effect on suicide. Risk increases with the size of families.
○ Resulted from an individual's insufficient integration within the society.
○ Durkheim concluded that it is our social rather than psychological sense which contributes to suicide.

4) *Altruistic suicide*
○ Persons in primitive societies who kill themselves because it is their duty (e.g. old people, followers upon the death of their superiors).

5) *Anomic suicide*
○ Resulted from excessive integration within the society to which one belongs.
○ When society is disturbed by crisis, society is temporarily incapable of exercising its regulatory function and the resulting lack of constraints makes happiness impossible.
○ This explains why countries in long-term poverty may have a low level of suicide but those experiencing sudden prosperity may have high levels.
○ *Anomie* – temporary condition of social deregulation.
○ *Anomic suicide* – self-inflicted death resulting from Anomie.

6) *Suicide as a social phenomenon*
○ At any moment, the degree of integration or regulation of a society determines its suicide rate.
○ When social conditions fail to provide people with the necessary objective or regulations, the most vulnerable in the society might commit suicide.

Michel Foucault (1926–1984)

• French philosopher.
• Work relevant to psychiatry includes several volumes on medicine and madness, as well as power resulting from discourse.

Medicine and madness

- 'Social constructionist' approach – 'external reality' does not exist. Our notions of body and health depend on discourses and how people see themselves.
- Foucault regarded mental illnesses as phenomena explicable only in terms of personal existence and of the meaning of the world perceived by the relevant individuals in imagination.
- Mental illness is the blocking of expression by a social system that prevents some people from acting on what they desire. Hence, therapy must help the person to move their social situation to one that allows such expression.
- Foucault's moral evaluation of madness: 4 key characteristics of classical madness:
  - included in the category of 'unreason'.
  - conceptually excluded from the life of 'reason'.
  - morally condemned as 'original choice' of unreason over reason.
  - perceived as an issue requiring administrative control.
- Madness distinguished from other unreasonableness by its 'animality'. Hence, the mentally ill can only be physically forced to obey.
- In the mid-18th century 'houses of confinement' were used for the 'mad', criminals and debtors. Madness became linked to moral fault.
- The public recognised it was wrong to house the 'mad' with criminals. This led to the establishment of the asylum.
- Foucault claimed that modern psychology and psychiatry depend fundamentally on the structure of asylum life.
- Doctors exert their power not by their medical knowledge, but by their moral authority.
- '*Gaze*' – the way of seeing and understanding that becomes synonymous with the thing itself.
- 'Medical gaze' – the 'medical gaze' of a doctor is a covert way of making moral judgement. 'Medical treatment' is merely a way of bringing the mad under the values of the bourgeois.
- Often, things we take for granted often result from our fabrication of discourses. Discourses often act as a source of power.
- His study of asylum and penal policy found that mental health and penal systems have become more controlling rather than more humane.

Discourse

- Foucault charts the social control from physical coercion to a more diffuse form of social surveillance and the process of 'normalisation'.
- An example is the Bentham's Panopticon (prison in which cells were arranged around a single watchtower from which a watchman could watch inmates, but the prisoners were never sure whether they were being watched).
- Discourse is the way in which certain subject matters are talked about in different social settings. There are often unspoken underlying assumptions to these discourses.
- Foucault pointed out how some types of discourses are preferred and become dominant. Other alternative types of discourses are marginalised.
- Such dominant discourses are often automatically perceived as 'true' and this is a source of power.
- Dominant discourses in different settings (e.g. schools, workplaces, society) determine our social or personal identity.

Talcott Parsons (1902–1979)

- School of structural-functionalism.
- How could there be any order if individuals pursue self-interests?
- Function – way of describing any given pattern of social interaction for the stability of the systems of interactions.
- These patterns contribute to the society's stability.
- A system has boundaries, interdependent parts and a tendency towards equilibrium.

Action systems

- Consist of cultural systems (for pattern maintenance), personality systems (for goal attainment), behavioural organisms (for adaptation) and social systems (for integration).
- Interrelations between the 4 systems:
  - *Internalisation* of social objects and cultural norms into the personality of the individual.
  - *Institutionalisation* – cultural and social systems are organised and stored in individual memory.

Social system

Structure of social systems may be analysed in terms of 4 components:

o values – defines desirable types of social systems. Important in maintaining patterns.
o norms – include both values and specific modes of orientation for acting under particular conditions of particular collectivities.
o collectivities – (there must be clear definition of membership and differentiation amongst its members) for attaining goals.
o roles – class of individuals involved in a particular collectivity. For example, during socialisation, education and learning, norms and values of society are internalised. Self interest and collective interests may conflict in any actions.

Society

o A self-sufficient collectivity with differentiation, segmentation and specification.
o *Differentiation* – e.g. kinship (according to sex, age, etc.).
o Power is the capacity to influence the allocation of resources for the goals for the collectivity.
o Authority consists of rules governing the making of specific binding decisions.
o *Segmentation* – relevant structures located at different levels.
o *Stratification* – legitimise differential power and wealth (e.g. social class stratification).

Goffman (1922–1982, Canadian)

• Relied mainly on observations and ethnographic methods to explain contemporary life.
• Started with the assumption that every facet of human behaviour is important.
• Total institutions
  o Goffman tried to avoid the bias inherent in the existing language about mental hospitals by using non-judgemental descriptive language and using words usually with negative connotations in a neutral way.
  o The time and interest people participated in it vary from a little to a lot. For some, it takes up almost all of the participants' lives and time 'total institutions'.

o The daily activity of a large number of persons is managed in a limited space with little resources.
o The rationales vary: 'good for people' (e.g. religious institutions), mortification (e.g. in penal system), and preparation for the self (e.g. military organisation).
o A division of labour between those who work towards laudable goals (e.g. senior doctors) and those who do the dirty work (e.g. attendants).
o Normal spheres of home, work and leisure are collapsed into one homogeneous social experience.
o Severance of relations outside and enter into new social relations inside.
o 3 aspects of a career in total institutions (e.g. mental hospitals)
   ▪ Mortification of the Self – loss of previous identity (e.g. removal of normal clothings).
   ▪ Reorganisation of the Self – aspects of identity with those of the hospital (e.g. hospital clothes).
   ▪ Patients' response – colonisation (acceptance without enthusiasm), conversion (identification with their new position) or withdrawn (rejection of hospital requirements).
   ▪ Compliance is rewarded with 'good patient' image. Negative sanctions may result from rejection of authority.
o Goffman's theory that the hospital environment may give rise to institutional neurosis was supported by a subsequent study of female patients with schizophrenia by Wing and Brown (1970).
o Tobin and Lieberman (1976) argued that for old people placed in nursing homes, loss of self-identity began before their physical removal.

Habermas (1929–)

• A member of the Frankfurt School of Critical theory.
• Disagreed with Marxism as it does not explain the lack of freedom in modern society.
• 'Crisis' occurs when modern society does not meet individual needs and institutions manipulate individuals.
• People respond to the crisis by 'communication action'.
• Theory of communication action
   o power is the key of communicative rationality
   o uses all human ways of thinking and language
   o allows human beings to understand and agree with one another

The agencies of socialisation

- Socialisation – the process whereby individuals learn the norms and values of the groups to which they belong and to prepare themselves for social interaction.
- The individual internalises these values through repeated actions.
- The process continues throughout life.
- Agencies of socialisation
  - Primary socialisation – includes the parents/guardians, the family or first carers.
  - Secondary socialisation – by other 'agents of socialisation', such as schools, the mass media, and religious organisations.
- Socialisation is a not a 1-way process. E.g. children are socialised by parents but can cause their parents to change, thus affecting their parents' socialisation.

Studies of community, kinship, marriage and the family

- Family forms differ considerably both historically and cross-culturally.
- Types of families
  - *Kinship groups* – groups made up of people who are related by blood or marriage.
  - *Nuclear family* – a household unit with a man and a woman in a stable marital relationship, together with their dependent children.
  - *Single-parent family* – a household unit with only 1 parent (usually the mother) residing with the children.
  - *Extended family* – a household unit with people from 3 or more generations.
  - *Reconstituted family* – a household unit with 1 or more step-parents as a result of previous divorce and marriage.
- Parsons' theory of a fit between industrial society and nuclear family
  - Economic differentiation compatible with nuclear but not extended families. Nuclear family avoids potential conflicts between members of an extended family working in different jobs, and is small enough to be geographically and economically mobile.
  - Families are characterised by values such as ascription (emphasis on who people are) and particularism (priority for special relationships).

Systems of social stratification

- Different systems of inequalities or stratifications exist in different historical and social contexts.
- Slavery – during periods of colonisation of Eastern countries by the West.
- Castes and estates – originated in the past when agriculture dominated the economics. Some elements have carried over to present-day societies.
- Class systems – predominate in modern industrial societies.

An estate system

- Based on land or an entity which controls the distribution of land (e.g. monarchy).
- Prevalent in Europe from the collapse of the Roman Empire to Industrial Revolution in 18th century.
- Most Eastern Asian countries (e.g. China, Japan) had an estate system until the 19th century.
- 3 estates: landed gentry, the clergy, the peasantry.
- *Landed gentry* – take control of the land and make decisions.
- *Clergy* – provide for the spiritual needs of the countryside.
- *Peasantry* – bottom of the hierarchy. Work on the land, provide goods and services for the gentry.

A caste system

- Existed in India and Nigeria.
- Also based in agriculture and ownership of property.
- Also distinguished between groups of people by their religious standing.
- Caste usually determined at birth with no opportunity of moving into other castes.
- Castes determine who individuals can marry, where they can live and the type of work they can do.
- The dominant caste has control of the society and how it is run.

A class system

- Ranking of individuals based on their economic power.
- Governed by several factors including income, wealth and occupation.

- May also be governed by how people do their job, irrespective of their income. E.g.
  - 'Upper class' – people who command others to work (e.g. managers) or rely on income or inheritance.
  - 'Working class' – people performing manual labour.
  - 'Middle class' – people performing clerical work or work involving primarily thinking.
  - 'Lower class' or 'underclass' – people with no steady or recognised jobs.

Theories of stratification

Marxist theory

See Marx above.

Weber's theory of bureaucracy

- A hierarchical system of authority based on an explicit set of rules.
- Theoretically allows efficient running of an organisation (e.g. hospital).
- Features include
  - Clear hierarchy of positions.
  - Explicit functions of each position.
  - Staff appointed on a contract.
  - Staff selection based on professional qualifications and examinations.
  - Salary based on hierarchy.
  - Post is the holder's only or main job.
  - Clear career structure, promotion based on merit perceived by superiors.
  - Staff subject to disciplinary procedures.

Social classes and inequality

Social class

Marx's theory of property relations

- Although industrialisation brought about wealth, it did so unequally.
- Bourgeoisie – control the means of production and monopolises the profits.

- Working Proletariat class – made poorer due to a tendency to keep wages at an exploitatively low level.
- Class conflict is inevitable with capitalism, as capitalism intends to exploit workers to raise profits.

Weber's theory of market relations

- There are 3 forms of inequalities: class, status and power.
- Those privileged in one form can use it to gain advantage in another.
- Weber focused on both access to occupations and property.

Class and inequality

- Registrar General's social class classification introduced in 1911 to analyse infant mortality rate
  - ○ I – Professional.
  - ○ II – Managerial and technical occupation.
  - ○ IIIN – Skilled non-manual.
  - ○ IIIM – Skilled manual.
  - ○ IV – Semi-skilled.
  - ○ V – Unskilled.
- Revised since then to take into account changes in occupational structure.
- Mortality and morbidity consistently shown to be highest in social class V and lowest in class I.
- Such inequalities in health officially reported in Black Report, and have persisted.
- Possible explanations of inequalities
  - ○ Labelling.
    - ■ Disease labels may be socially constructed.
    - ■ E.g. those in the lower social classes are more likely to be labelled as mentally ill (Scheff).
  - ○ Doctors may misinterpret cultural beliefs.
  - ○ Social selection.
    - ■ Include both downward social drift and poor health preventing upward drift.
    - ■ Goldberg and Morrison (1963) – found over twice as many patients with schizophrenia in social class V at admission than expected by chance. However, difference disappears if social class were defined by fathers' occupations at the time of birth.

○ Provision of medical services.
  ■ Access and quality of medical services may be lower for lower social class.
  ■ Unlikely to be a major cause for health inequalities, as many conditions are not amenable to treatment.
○ Life-style
  ■ Those in lower social classes may engage in high-risk lifestyles such as smoking, high alcohol consumption or low fibre diet.
○ Environmental risk.
  ■ Those in lower social classes may be exposed to environments with higher risks to health (e.g. exposure to smoke, asbestos, overcrowding).
○ Lack of material resources.
  ■ Poverty is an important factor.
  ■ E.g. lack of nutritious food, accident preventing equipment.
  ■ E.g. lack of social network.

Reproduction of social class

According to Weber, social class tends to pass on from one generation by

- Social closure – efforts made by social groups to protect their own interest by denying outsiders from entering the group.
- Social reproduction – the process by which groups of people pass on their social structures and patterns to future generations (e.g. through ability to pay for private education).

Social mobility

- The movement of individuals from one position in the social hierarchy (e.g. social class, occupational position) to another.
- May be within a generation (intragenerational) or between generations (intergenerational mobility).
- 3 main factors affecting social mobility
  ○ *Changing number of positions to be filled* – in the last 20 years, marked decline in manufacturing jobs and a shift towards service-sector jobs, which particularly suit women.
  ○ *Methods of access and entry to these positions* – qualifications and skills have become more important. However, children from middle-class parents, ethnic minorities and disabled people are at a disadvantage even with the same level of education.

- *Number of suitable offspring available to fill the positions* – for example, 25% of professional and managerial staff in the UK are drawn from the working class as there are not sufficient middle-class young people with appropriate qualifications to fill the posts.
- Strong evidence of a glass ceiling for women in getting professional and managerial positions in the past, but the gender difference has now narrowed considerably.
- Affected by changing structure of labour market
  - Growth of part-time jobs causes a large increase in women workers.
  - Reduction of secure lifelong positions increases risk of downward mobility.

Social change in the modern world

How modernity originates

Modernity started around the late 19th century when complex and enormous social, economical, political, cultural and technological changes began to emerge and marked a distinct break from the traditional ways of life.

- *More efficient forms of production*: new ways of working caused by industrialisation and division of labour.
- *Capitalism*: the rise of new financial institutions and entrepreneurship in pursuit of profits, market economy, the treatment of labour, goods and services as commodities.
- *Population and demographic changes*: exponential increase in population, mass movement of people from rural to urban areas (i.e. urbanisation), migration across countries.
- *New forms of governments*: development of bureaucratic organisations, emergence of new political ideas (e.g. citizenship, nationalism).
- *Western expansion and colonisation*: sometimes leads to economic prosperity for western countries but destruction of societies in other countries.

Social changes associated with modernism

- *Industrialisation*
  - Large scale factory system.
  - Clock-driven.

- o Takes place outside home.
- o Division of labour – specialised tasks for workers.
- o Development of hierarchy of labour based on skills.
- o Rise of trade unions to fight for better working conditions.
- o Employers attempt to get the most from their workforce.
- *Capitalism*
  - o Emergence of market system and 'consumerism' – a culture based on promotion and sales of goods.
  - o Products valued for their novelty and creativity.
- *Rationality*
  - o Weber – modernity results from the pre-occupation of using the most efficient ways to achieve one's goal.
  - o E.g. economies of scale, assembly-line production.
  - o Rationality is the purpose of bureaucratic organisations.
  - o Associated with rise of science, industrialisation, capitalism (efficient pursuit of profits), and codified law (rational organisation of justice).
- *Increased expectation of technology*
  - o Uses: e.g. medical technologies and computers.
  - o Misuses: e.g. nuclear or chemical warfare.
- *Increased government control*
  - o Occurs in most forms of government (e.g. democratic, communist).
  - o Via both compulsion and consent.
  - o E.g. codified legal system, control over economic systems, national systems of education and welfare.

The concepts of conformity and deviance

Lemert's social reaction theory

- Deviance – behaviour once known publicly is subjected to sanctions.
- Primary deviance – an undesirable difference from the norm.
- Secondary deviance – an individual reorganises his or her own perception to match socially defined expectations.

Social construction of illness and deviance (Parsons' model)

- Sick role (see below).

Social construction of illness and deviance (Freidson's model)

	Illegitimate (i.e. stigmatised)	Conditionally legitimate (if compliant)	Unconditionally legitimate
Minor deviation	E.g. mild deafness; some ordinary obligations partially suspended; few new privileges, few new obligations	E.g. acute back pain; few ordinary obligations suspended temporarily; ordinary privileges enhanced, obligations to seek treatment	E.g. large facial moles; no changes in obligations or privileges
Major deviation	E.g. mentally ill; some ordinary obligations suspended; some new obligations imposed; few new privileges	E.g. septicaemia; ordinary obligations temporarily suspended; additional ordinary privileges, obligations to seek treatment	E.g. malignancies; ordinary obligations suspended permanently, many new privileges

Labelling behaviour

- Deviance is a label assigned to individuals by people in authority.
- Provides a source of power to those in a position to put labels on individuals.
- What is considered to be deviant varies with time and situation.
- Durkheim
  - Anomie – state of normlessness in society. People unclear what is expected of them.
  - Anomie theory – deviant behaviour is encouraged by strains inherent in society.
- Merton (1956)
  - 4 ways in which people adapt to stress: conformity, innovation, ritualism, rebellion.
- Scheff (1966)
  - Formal labelling (e.g. mental illness, HIV) can be stigmatising.
  - 'Labelling is the most important cause of mental illness'.

- Behaviour may be classified as a sign of mental illness and referred to official agencies depending on the reaction of others to the act of 'residual rule breaking' (i.e. breaking of unspecified rules of conduct expected to be followed in social situations).
- Likelihood of residual rule-breaking being referred to an official agency depends on
  - Perceived seriousness of the act.
  - Level of tolerance of residual rule-breaking in the community.
  - The social distance between rule-breaker and the controlling agents. Chance of referral is greater if rule-breaker is of low social status.

Responses of those stigmatised (Goffman)

- Goffman distinguished between discreditable (i.e. not immediately visible or known) and discrediting (i.e. visible) attributes.
- Possible reactions
  - Attempt to correct defects (e.g. plastic surgery).
  - Accept defects.
  - Unconventional reactions (e.g. use for secondary gain, excuse for failure in unrelated areas).
- Reactions to discreditable attributes
  - Passing – attempt to conceal (e.g. artificial aids), but may be stressful for stigma bearer.
  - Covering – attempt to reduce its significance (e.g. by reducing visibility of the defects).
  - Withdrawal – opting out of social activities.

Anspach's strategy for managing stigma

Depends on the self-image of the stigma bearer and whether they accept the dominant social values

	Accept social value	Reject social value
Positive self-image	Normalisation	Political activism – seek to repudiate social values
Negative self-image	Disassociation	Retreatism

Impairment, disability and handicap

- Impairment – mechanical deviation from the norm.
- Disability – reduced performance due to impairment.
- Handicap – disadvantage resulting from an impairment or disability (i.e. social phenomenon).

Social causes of illness

Social support

- Socio-environmental approach to disease – social factors contribute to the risk of disease through increasing physiological risk factors (e.g. hypertension), behavioural risks (e.g. poor diet or smoking) and psychosocial risk factors (e.g. lack of social support).
- Durkheim (1897) found that high rates of suicide were associated with groups with very high or very low levels of social integration.
- Married people have lower mortality rates than single, widowed and divorced people.
- Berkman and Syme (1979) found those with low social networks have 2–3 × higher mortality rates.
- Brown and Harris (1978) – social support protects against depression only in the context of a severe life event.

Life events

- Holmes and Rahe (1967) developed the Social Readjustment Rating Scale (SRRS). Studies found some relationship between life events and future health.
- Criticisms of these studies: ignores less severe life difficulties, did not take into account significance of life events.
- Brown and Harris (1978)
  - Clear relationship between onset of depression in women and life events with long-term threatening implications.
  - However, no relationship with life events with only short-term implications.
- Life events may be associated with physical and functional disorders.

Concepts of adversity and resilience

Resilience

- The capacity to withstand and overcome adversity; the capacity to moderate physiological and external events such as life events.
- Graded rather than all-or-none phenomenon.
- Changes with circumstances and not an individual's intrinsic trait.
- Characteristics (Rutter)
  - Originates from exposure to risk rather than avoidance of risk factors.
  - May stem from early life experiences.
  - A risk factor may be protective in one situation but harmful in another.
- 3 models on the impact of stress and personal attitudes on adaptation (Garmezy, Masten and Tellegen)
  - Compensatory model – competence increases with reduced stress and increased personal resilience. Linear relationship between stress and competence.
  - Challenge model – Moderate amount of stress increases competence. Inverted U-shaped relationship between stress and competence.
  - Conditional model – Personal attributes modify the impact of stress on competence.
- Examples of risk mechanisms and buffering factors
  - Adult social support buffers against the effects of parental divorce on children's adjustment.
- Rutter outlined 4 different protective mechanisms
  - Reducing risk impact.
  - Reducing negative chain reactions.
  - Establishing and maintaining self-esteem.
  - Establishing and maintaining self-efficacy.
- Maternal criticism and child development
  - Maternal criticism is associated with child behavioural inhibition, other behavioural disorders and mood disorders.
  - Maternal emotional over-involvement is associated with child separation anxiety disorder.
- Expressed emotion (EE)
  - Term first used by Brown *et al.* 1972.
  - An index of characteristics in relatives likely to be associated with a florid relapse of schizophrenia.

o High EE families have a high level of criticism, intrusion and verbal output.
o EE is the single best predictor of relapse in schizophrenia during the first 9 months following discharge from hospital.
o EE is a strong predictor in patients with more longstanding illness but not in a first-episode patient.

History of UK health services from 20th century

• 1911 – Lloyd George introduced compulsory insurance for poor manual workers, but non-workers had to pay for health care.
• First and second world war – recruitment to wars revealed prevalence of poor health.
• 1942 – Beveridge Commission Report suggested national health service.
• 1948
  o NHS Act came into place.
  o Overriding aim – to provide free health services to all those in need, from cradle to grave.
  o Health service cost funded from taxes.
  o GPs contracted with NHS to retain autonomy.
  o Consultants salaried.
  o Largest employer.
• 1948–1977 – Tripartite model
  o General practitioners, hospitals, local authorities.
  o Hospital Management Committees.
  o Porritt Report (1962) criticised separation of NHS into 3 parts and called for unification.
  o Became unsustainable in 1974 due to unwillingness of GPs to participate and better administration required for hospitals.
• 1974–1982 – Consensus model
  o Area and District Health Authorities established, in addition to Regional Health Authorities
  o Decision made by agreement between all parties.
  o Doctors had clinical autonomy.

- o Sir Roy Griffiths reported that this was inefficient and advised general management style as in other private corporations.
- 1982–1990 – General Management model
  - o NHS costs continued to escalate.
  - o General managers at hospitals.
  - o From 1983 – Line management model with accountability at every level.
  - o Doctors' clinical autonomy threatened.
  - o 1989 White Paper 'Working for Patients' suggested the internal market model.
- 1990–1997
  - o NHS and Community Care Act.
  - o Internal market system to address problems (e.g. long waiting list).
  - o NHS Trusts set up between 1991 and 1995. They are independent entities with their own management and financial budgets.
  - o Purchasers (i.e. Health Authorities and Fundholding GPs) and providers (i.e. NHS Trust and non-fundholding GPs).
  - o Purchasers contracted with providers to buy services according to specifications.
  - o Aimed to introduce competition and to improve quality of services.
  - o Also aimed to increase patients' choices.
  - o When Labour Government came into power in 1997, internal market was thought to result in unnecessary duplication of services.
  - o White Paper 'The New NHS: Modern, Dependable' put forward a third way of running the service based on partnership and driven by performance.
  - o 6 principles of the White Paper: ensure fair access, local responsibility, working in partnerships, increase efficiency, focus on quality of care and rebuild public confidence.
- 1997–Current
  - o Regional Health Authority downsized and replaced by Regional Offices.
  - o Health Authority responsibilities gradually taken over by Primary Care Trust, each covering about a population of 100,000.
  - o Salaried GPs introduced.
  - o Clinical governance proposed.
  - o Revalidation of doctors proposed.

Different cultural models of illness and their impact on illness behaviour

- Consultation rates vary depending on sex, age, social class and ethnic groups
  - Women consulted more often than men.
  - Extremes of age (older people and children) consult more often than other age groups.
  - Ethnic minorities consult GPs more often but use hospital services less.
- The decision to consult depends on how patients respond to their symptoms.
- Mechanic's variables known to influence illness behaviour
  - Visibility of signs and symptoms.
  - Person's perception of seriousness of symptoms.
  - Extent to which symptoms affect family, work or social life.
  - Frequency, persistence and recurrence of symptoms.
  - Available information and level of understanding of these symptoms.
  - Other competing needs which may lead a person to ignore symptoms.
  - Other possible explanations for the symptoms and signs.
  - Availability of health professionals and the monetary and psychological costs of seeking help.
- Cultural variation in illness behaviour
  - E.g. Anglo-Saxon patients tend to withstand pain in a matter-of-fact fashion while Mediterranean patients tend to seek help.
  - Asian patients may tend to attribute physical problems to psychological symptoms.

The social role of medicine and the sociology of professions

Parsons' model of the sick role and the doctor's role

Doctor's social role	Patient's sick role
Obligations	
1. Provide a high standard of professional services	1. Must seek professional medical advice

2. Act in the personal interest of the patient
3. Act objectively and in non-judgemental way
4. Abide by professional regulations

Privileges

1. Take appropriate history and perform physical examination
2. Significant autonomy in professional work
3. In a position of authority

2. Must co-operate with health professionals and aim to recover as soon as possible

1. Relieved of usual responsibilities (e.g. housework or employment)
2. Considered to be in need of care in order to get better.

Possible conflicts in doctor's role

- Doctors need to act both in the patient's interest and in the interest of the state as gatekeepers to the sick role (e.g. issue of sick notes).
- Individual patient's interest competing with public interest (e.g. rationing of health resources).
- Confidentiality issues (e.g. epileptic patients who insist on driving).

Stewart and Roter's doctor–patient relationship matrix

	Doctor's control low	Doctor's control high
Patient's control low	Default	Paternalism
Patient's control high	Consumerism	Mutuality

Parson's model generally assumes a paternalist relationship. There is a general shift from paternalism to consumerism or mutuality over time.

Sociology of professions

- Characteristics of professions (Goode)
  - Profession determines its own standard of training.
  - Lengthy training in an accredited institution.
  - Body of specialised knowledge.
  - Monopoly of their field of work (e.g. by state registration).

- o Admission and licensing processes are run by the professions.
- o Autonomy to organise and develop their work.
- o Codes of ethics.
- o Usually under social class I or II, high power and status.
- o Practitioners relatively free of lay evaluation and control.
- o Usually a life-time occupation for practitioners.
- Process of selection to professions.
- Involve acquisition of relevant knowledge, appropriate attitudes and behaviour towards clients and colleagues.

Sex and gender differences

A continuum of approaches to explain sex or gender differences

- Biological determinism – differences explained simply in terms of biological or genetic characteristics.
- Masculinity and femininity – socially constructed sets of assumptions, expectations and behaviour associated with and assigned to men/women in a specific culture.
- Essentialism – an approach assuming all women share traits in common, as for men.

Differences between sex and gender

- Sex – biological differences between men and women (e.g. in terms of chromosomes, genitalia, reproductive capacity). Usually dichotomous.
- Gender – Difference in social and cultural meanings attached to males and females.

Acquiring gender

- By 2 years of age, most children acquire a gender identity (sense of themselves as either male or female).
- Gender identity does not necessarily correspond to biological sex (e.g. transsexuals).

- Socialisation theory – from interaction with others, infants learn the sex attributed to them by positive or negative reinforcement. Cannot explain the complexity of gender identity and desires.
- Chodorow's psychoanalytic theory
  - Mothers usually care for their infants, while fathers are more distant.
  - Formation of self depends on separation with the mother with whom the infant is initially psychically merged.
  - Girls usually separate with mothers gradually, maintaining a continuous relationship.
  - Boys separate from their mother and repress their feminine aspects.
  - Explains why men have more difficulty in expressing emotions and intimacy.
  - Explains why women have the natural abilities of childcare.

Social roles

- *Before industrialisation* in 1780s, all household members worked irrespective of age and sex.
- *From 1780s*, industrialisation separated the places of home and work.
- Ideology of domesticity (i.e. women's roles to look after home) dominated.
- Division of labour by gender: men perceived to be more rational and women more emotional.
- Women were barred from higher education and higher levels of employment. Women entered high social class by marrying wealthy men.
- However, women's contributions (e.g. housework, carers) were often forgotten.
- *From 1950s*, more women entered employment due to
  - shift from manufacturing to service industry.
  - expansion in employment.
- However, inequalities between men and women still existed
  - Horizontal gender segregation – separation of men and women into qualitatively different types of jobs. E.g. more men as professionals (e.g. medical or legal professions) and as labourers, more women as nurses, secretaries and cleaners.
  - Vertical gender segregation – separation of men and women into higher or lower grades within the same occupation (e.g. existence of glass ceilings for women managers).

Patriarchy

- An overarching system of male dominance in society, often with dominance of senior men over both women and junior men.
- Walby's 6 discrete structures of patriarchy
  - Role of men in households.
  - Organisation of paid work.
  - Patriarchal state.
  - Male violence.
  - Heterosexuality and the sexual double standard (i.e. men's place to initiate sex and women's responsibility to decide how far a sexual encounter should go).
  - Cultural institutions and practices.
- Walby's 2 types of patriarchy
  - *Private patriarchy* – focus on the ideology of domesticity. Household production as the crucial structure. Women controlled by husbands and fathers. Dominated before 19th century.
  - *Public patriarchy* – occurs with entry of women into labour force. Women controlled collectively through employment practices.
- Connell's theory of gender order – definitions of masculinities and femininities have 4 separate elements.
  - Labour – organisation of employment, housework and childcare.
  - Power – association of masculinity with authority.
  - Cathexis – social and psychological patterning of desire and the construction of emotionally charged relationships.
  - Symbolism – symbolic structures used in communication.

Race inequalities, racism and racial harassment

Race and ethnicity

- Race – biological differences based on skin colour.
- Ethnicity – sense of belonging to a particular community sharing a particular culture.

Race inequalities and legal responses

- In Europe, partly related to history of colonialism.
- Also related to mass migration of people from the Commonwealth in the 1950s due to staff shortages caused by economic boom.
- Proportion of ethnic minorities in the UK was 0.4% in 1950, 2.3% in 1970 and 5.5% in 1990.
- In 1950s, open racial discrimination was lawful. Non-whites filled jobs that others did not want.
- Immigration issues become and remain highly political – e.g. Nottingham and Notting Hill race riots in 1958, demonstrations and race-motivated murder of Stephen Lawrence in 1990s.
- Immigration Acts in 1960s and 1970s restricted immigration from the Commonwealth, particularly for black people.
- With economic recession in late 1970s, ethnic minorities were at much greater risk of unemployment.
- Race Relations Act (1976) was passed due to political unacceptability of clear disadvantages faced by immigrants. Intended to outlaw discrimination on racial grounds in employment matters.
- It was only partially effective because it was difficult for anyone claiming discrimination to prove that it was on racial grounds.
- The Race Relations (Amendment) Act 2000 makes it unlawful to discriminate against anyone on grounds of race, colour, nationality or ethnicity.

Current race inequalities

Recent independent research by Policy Studies Institute found

- Racial discrimination and harassment affect all ethnic minority groups.
- Bangladeshis and Pakistanis are the poorest people in the UK.
- Serious under-representation of all minorities in top 10% of all jobs.
- Black and Asian people have lower paid jobs than whites with the same education and skills.

The Institute for Social and Economic Research found

- Young Afro-Caribbean men were more than twice as likely to be out of work than corresponding white men.
- Bangladeshi and Pakistani men were more likely to be unemployed than corresponding Afro-Caribbean men.

Areas other than employment

- People from ethnic minorities have inferior housing compared to Whites.
- Black people tend to have poorer access to social service provisions.

Use of health services

- Generally, ethnic minority groups had higher utilisation of GP services, but their utilisation of outpatient services was lower.
- Black people are twice as likely to be compulsorily admitted to psychiatric hospital as the general population. There are disputes on whether this is due to different thresholds of diagnosing psychosis by psychiatrists or to increased incidence of mental illness.
- Ethnic minorities were more likely than the general population to perceive the quality of primary care service as lower in some respects, especially for Bangladeshis and Pakistanis. They were less likely to be happy with the outcome of the consultation overall.

Medical profession

Research by Kings Fund (2001) found

- Non-white doctors are at substantial disadvantages at all stages of their career, such as
  - entry to medical school.
  - application for senior house officer, registrar and consultant posts.
  - seeking discretionary points (extra payments that doctors can earn at the top of their career).
- A 'concrete wall effect' for non-White doctors to progress up the career ladder.
- Daily harassment of black and Asian doctors.

Impact of racism

- Institute of Race Relations (2001) reported
  - over 23,000 racist incidents of violence.
  - 28 racially motivated murders in England and Wales between 1999 and 2001.
- Public enquiries uncovered prevalence of *institutional racism* (i.e. implicit, taken for granted, reproduction of racism by institutions), including police and NHS.

- Racist beliefs are shared cultural phenomena, not merely confined to deviant individuals.
- Discrimination is much more likely to be covert than overt.
- Stereotype of refugees or asylum seekers as economic immigrants.

New racism

- Described by Baker 1981.
- 'New form of racism based on ideas of cultural difference rather than on claims of biological superiority'.
- Characteristics
  - Claims that current significance of racism is exaggerated.
  - Defines groups as cultural communities rather than biological types.
  - Denies that hostility towards other groups is racist, but argues that it is natural for people to wish to be with their own group.
  - Justifies preferential treatment of one group over another based on their differences rather than superiority.

Migration and mental illness

- Immigrants generally have a higher level of mental illness than both native-born population and the population where they originate.
- E.g. West Indians have high prevalence rates of schizophrenia.
- Cox – 3 hypothesis to explain association between migration and mental illness
  - Selection hypothesis – certain mental disorders make the sufferers migrate.
  - Stress hypothesis – process of migration precipitates mental illness.
  - Confounding variables – e.g. age, class, cultural conflicts.
- Selection hypothesis
  - Restless and unstable people may be more likely to migrate more often.
  - Some evidence – e.g. half of non-British female immigrants to Australia who developed mental illness within 3 years had previous episodes before their migration.
  - Unlikely to be the only explanation.
- Stress hypothesis
  - E.g. overcrowding, shared accommodation, unemployment, low income, racial discrimination, language difficulties.
  - Factors affecting stress response: individuals' characteristics, physical environment, social support, economic status, cultural background.

Special problems for refugees

- Many have experienced acts of extreme violence.
- 'Cultural bereavement' – grief for loss of everything that symbolises their origins.
- Many are confronted with hostility in their home countries.

Relationship between culture, society and psychiatry

Normality

- Physiological measurements less important in psychiatry.
- 'Culturally normal' – social definitions based on shared beliefs within a group of people as to what constitutes 'proper'.
- A multi-dimensional concept, including factors relating to the individual, social context and social relationship.
- Relevant individual factors: behaviour, dress, posture, gestures, facial expression, tone of voice, use of language.
- Some bizarre behaviour may be accepted if conform to implicit guidelines in a society (e.g. assertion of being possessed by supernatural forces).
- Same behaviour may be regarded as 'normal' in one situation if socially controlled, or 'mad' or 'bad' in a second if socially uncontrolled.
- Distinction between 'mad' and 'bad' may depend on perceived level of insight of the individual.

Comparing psychological disorders across cultures

Comparison may be problematic as disorders are socially defined.

Biological approach

- Kiev – views form of psychiatric disorders as constant and universal across the world.
- Tendency to classify disorders in other cultures within same classification as Western culture. E.g. Amok in Malaya as a dissociative state.
- 2 disadvantages: category fallacy (i.e. category in one cultural group may not apply to another culture) and it ignores the different social roles played by the same mental illness in different societies.

Social labelling approach

- Regard mental illness as a myth, as a social rather than biological fact.
- Waxler – mental illness is defined relevant to the society.
- Consists of 2 stages: labelling after a minor deviant behaviour and individuals subsequently playing the role.
- Labelling: risk of being labelled depends on individual's power relative to labeller (e.g. age, sex, race, social class).
- Once labelled, a number of cultural cues tell the individual how to play their role.
- Individuals then depend on society to re-label them.

Combined approach

- Recognises certain universal abnormal behaviours (e.g. psychosis).
- Also recognises wide variation in the form and geographical distribution of mental disorders.
- More valid to compare symptom patterns than diagnostic categories.

Factors influencing psychiatric diagnosis

- Relatively few tests on biological malfunction compared to physical disorders.
- Mostly depend on doctors' subjective evaluation, as few patients possess the entire typical cluster of symptoms.
- Doctors' factors: personality, experience, length of diagnostic interview, style of interview, social class, ethnic, cultural and religious background in relation to patients.
- Moral considerations: e.g. whether doctors consider alcoholism as 'ill', 'mad' or 'bad'.
- Szasz argued that diagnosis may be politically motivated (e.g. labelling political dissenters as mad).
- Black people are more likely to be diagnosed as having drug-induced psychosis by UK psychiatrists than Whites.
- UK-born Afro-Caribbeans are 9 times more likely to be diagnosed with schizophrenia, although this may also be partly due to social and economic disadvantages.

History of psychiatry

History of psychiatry from antiquity to the present day

From 1500 BC to 1200 AD

- 1500 BC – early Egyptian papyri contain references to mental disturbances.
- Ancient Greek – record of mania, melancholia and paranoia associated with physical illnesses.
- Hippocrates in 400 BC – regarded mental illnesses as requiring medical treatment.

From 12th to 18th century AD

- Mental illnesses often regarded as a spiritual rather than a medical problem.
- E.g. Jurors returned a verdict of misadventure when they found that the accused was acting under *'the instigation of the devil'* and that his illness had rendered him *'frantic and mad'* and thus susceptible to 'the wiles of Satan'.
- 1188 – Henry II bought land close to Newgate as a prison, where the Old Bailey now stands.
- 1247 – Bethlem Hospital, first hospital for the insane, was founded.
- 1290 – De Prerogative Regis ('The King's Perogative') – a statute giving the King custody of the lands of 'natural fools' while they were insane.
- 1403 there were only 6 insane and 3 sane patients in Bethlem Hospital. Hospital found to be in a deplorable state for patients.
- 1547 – King Henry VIII gave Bethlem Hospital and St Bartholomew Hospital to the City of London (i.e. lay people).
- 1666 – Great fire of London. New Bethlem Hospital opened in 1676.
- 1695 – record of the public being allowed to view patients in the New Bethlem Hospital on payment of a fee.
- 1670 – private 'madhouses' set up. Detained people could apply to the Court for wrongful imprisonment.
- 1690 – Locke introduced ideas that madness is the inability to associate ideas correctly.
- 1714 Vagrancy Act – first English statute for detention of lunatics.

- 1749 – David Hartley linked 'association of ideas theory of human mind' to the nervous system.
- 1774 –Madhouses Act – licensed private madhouses, which were also routinely inspected. About 40 private small madhouses.
- Early 1770s – St Peter's Church used as a workhouse for boys, together with 'infants, the aged, infirm and lunatics'.
- 1788 – King George III suffered from recurrent mental disorder. King was removed to Kew for therapeutic confinement. His illness stimulated discussion about the treatment of mentally ill people.
- 1800 Criminal Lunatic Act – for safe custody of criminal lunatics.

The Modern era – late 18th century to 1910s

- 1828 – first professor of psychiatry in Germany.
- 1832 – St Peter's Hospital became a lunatic asylum.
- 1830–1860 – *General therapeutic optimism*. Belief that asylum treatment was the correct and scientific way of managing people with mental disorders. Move towards more humane (moral) treatment of the insane.
- 1841 – half of all doctors looking after mentally ill patients joined the asylum doctor association.
- 1844 – record of some asylums using non-restraint methods, while others used mechanical restraint of patients.
- 1860–1900 – *General therapeutic pessimism*. Morel's theory of degeneration – mental illness is the product of hereditary incurable degenerative disease and that asylum treatment could not cure the illness. By 1890s, patients were sent to even larger asylums only to protect them from society's exploitation and society from them.
- 1863 – Broadmoor Criminal Lunatic Asylum opened.
- 1890 Lunacy Act – private patients could not be detained without a judicial order from a Justice of the Peace specialising in such orders.
- 1910 – Rampton Hospital opened as the first state institution for mentally defective people who were considered dangerous.
- 1913 Mental Deficiency Act – built 'colonies' to separate the defectives from the gene pool of the rest of the population.

Significant events in 1910–1930

- *Psychoanalytic theories* – Freud's successful use of hypnosis and free association to treat patients with hysteria. Highlighted importance of psychological factors in aetiology and management.

- *First World War* – Shell-shock cases led to the understanding that exposure to untoward events may cause mental illness.
- *Trends in psychiatric treatment*
  - Away from asylum or inpatient treatment.
  - More out-patient treatment.
  - More informal treatment without 'certification'.

1930–present day

- 1930 Mental Treatment Act – made provisions for voluntary treatment and psychiatric outpatient treatment.
- Late 1940s – about 100 asylums each with 1,000 patients. Buildings were badly in need of repair.
- 1950s – cost of renovating the buildings caused governments to consider alternatives, such as community care.
- 1957 Percy Report – 2 key points
  - Mental disorder should be regarded in much the same way as physical disorders.
  - Hospitals for mental disorders should be run in much the same way as those for physical disorders.
- 1959 Mental Health Act based on the key points in the Percy Report.
- By 1959, only 12% of admissions were compulsory.
- 1970s – call for mentally handicapped people to lead their lives as close to normal as possible, and to integrate with the community.
- 1981 – White Paper 'Care in the Community' – move resources from NHS to local councils and voluntary organisations.
- 1990s – closure of large long-stay mental hospitals.

New types of treatment in the 20th century

- 1930s – insulin coma treatment for schizophrenia.
- 1938 – use of ECT for schizophrenia.
- 1949 – introduction of lithium salts.
- 1954 – use of chlorpromazine.
- 1957 – use of monoamine oxidase inhibitor antidepressants.
- 1958 – use of tricyclic antidepressants.
- 1964 – psychosurgery (e.g. leucotomy).
- 1970s – use of long-acting phenothiazines.

Models of madness

- Biomedical (somatic) model
  - View mental illness as a biological disease.
  - Focus on use of physical treatment (e.g. medication).
- Foucault
  - With the concern of the Enlightenment for reasons, large institutions emerged to house 'unreasonable' people.
  - The real purpose of these institutions was social exclusion.
  - Psychiatrists emerged as a result of the existence of these asylums rather than their ability to cure mental illness.
  - Psychiatry replaces spiritual and moral understanding of madness with a technological and scientific framework.
- Rosenhan (1973) – 'Pseudo-patients' were diagnosed with schizophrenia and gained admission to US psychiatric hospitals with a single false complaint of hearing a voice saying 'hollow' or 'empty'. These labels remained although the symptoms were never mentioned again.
- Illich – critiques medicalisation and put into doubt the value of doctors and psychiatrists.
- Antipsychiatrists
  - Szasz – exposes the use of psychiatry as a political tool for state repression and coercion.
  - Liang – "The experience and behaviour that gets labelled schizo-phrenic is a special strategy that a person invents in order to live in an unliveable situation".
- Mayer's bio-psychological model
  - Emphasis on the understanding of the person.
  - Mental illnesses are psychologically (rather than biologically) mediated.
  - Boundary between mentally normal and mentally ill is fluid be-cause normal people can become ill if exposed to sufficiently severe trauma.
  - Mental illness is viewed as a continuum – normal, neurosis, borderline conditions and psychosis.
- Post-psychiatry (Bracken and Thomas 2001)
  - Declining trust in the ability of science and technology to tackle human and social problems.
  - Post-psychiatry emphasises social and cultural contexts, places ethics before technology, and works to minimise medical control of coercive interventions.

Reading list

General

Johnstone EC. Companion to psychiatric studies. Edinburgh: Churchill Livingstone, 1998.

Leung WC, Passmore K. Essential Notes for MRCPsych Part I. Newbury: Petroc Press, 2001.

Neurosciences

Bear M, Connors B and Paradiso M. Neuroscience: exploring the brain, 2nd edition. Lippincott Williams and Wilkins, 2001.

Snell RS. Clinical neuroanatomy for medical students, 5th edition. Lippincott Williams and Wilkins, 2001.

Yudofsy and Hales. The American Psychiatric Press textbook of neuropsychiatry, 3rd edition. American Psychiatric Press, 1999.

Social sciences

Scambler G. Sociology as applied to medicine, 4th edition. London: WB Saunders, 1997.

Annandale E. The sociology of health and medicine: a critical introduction. Cambridge: Polity Press, 1998.

Macionis JJ. Sociology: a global introduction, 2nd edition. Harlow: Prentice Hall, 2002.

Epidemiology

Coggon D. Epidemiology for the uninitiated, 4th edition. London: BMJ, 1997.

Farmer RDT. Lecture notes on epidemiology and public health medicine, 4th edition. Oxford: Blackwell Science, 1996.

Tsuang MT and Tohen M. Textbook in psychiatric epidemiology, 2nd edition. New York: Wiley-Liss, 2002 (for reference only).

Statistics and research methods

Bland M. An introduction to medical statistics, 3rd edition. Oxford: Oxford University Press, 2000.

Genetics

Rimoin DL, Connor JM, Pyeritz, Korf BR and Emergy AE. Emergy and Rimoin's principles and practice of medical genetics, 4th edition. Edinburgh: Churchill Livingstone, 2002.

Neiderhiser JM. Understanding the roles of genome and envirome: methods in genetic epidemiology. British Journal of Psychiatry 2001; 178(suppl 40): s12–17.

Rutter M, Silberg J, O'Connor T and Simonoff E. Genetics and child psychiatry: I. Advances in quantitative and molecular genetics. Journal of Child Psychology and Psychiatry and Allied Disciplines 1999; 40(1): 3–18.

Rutter M, Silberg J, O'Connor T and Simonoff E. Genetics and child psychiatry: II. Empirical research findings. Journal of Child Psychology and Psychiatry and Allied Disciplines 1999; 40(1): 19–55.

Ethics and the law

Montgomery J. Health care law, 2nd edition. Oxford: Clarendon, 2003.

Macgregor-Morris R, Ewbank J and Birmingham L. Potential impact of the Human Rights Act on psychiatric practice: the best of British values? British Medical Journal 2001; 322: 848–850.